RENAL DIET COOKBOOK
FOR BEGINNERS 2024

The Complete Guide With 1900 Days of Life-Changing Low Potassium, Sodium, Phosphorus and Limited Protein Recipes to Manage Stage of Kidney Disease

4-Weeks Meal Plan Included

JUANITA SCOTT

DISCLAIMER

The information provided in this book is for general informational purposes only. It is not intended to be a substitute for professional medical advice, diagnosis, or treatment. Always seek the advice of your physician or other qualified health provider with any questions you may have regarding a medical condition.

The author and publisher of this book have made every effort to ensure that the information in this book is accurate and up-to-date at the time of publication. However, they make no representations or warranties of any kind, express or implied, about the completeness, accuracy, reliability, suitability, or availability of the information contained within. The author and publisher disclaim any responsibility for any adverse effects or consequences resulting from the use of the information presented in this book.

The dietary recommendations and recipes provided in this book are intended as general guidelines and may not be suitable for everyone. Individual nutritional needs vary, and it is advisable to consult with a qualified healthcare professional or registered dietitian before making significant changes to your diet.

This book may contain references to specific products, services, or third-party websites. These references are provided for informational purposes only and do not constitute an endorsement or recommendation.

JUANITA SCOTT

JUANITASCOTT007@GMAIL.COM

ABOUT THE AUTHOR

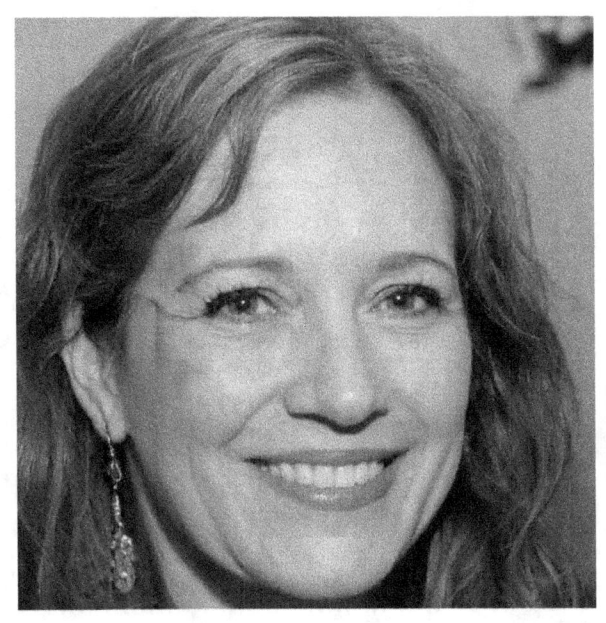

Meet Juanita Scott, a culinary virtuoso, seasoned nutritionist, and dedicated dietitian whose passion for healthy eating and lifestyle has transformed the lives of many. Beyond the artistry of the kitchen, Juanita brings a wealth of expertise, seamlessly blending her culinary mastery with a deep understanding of nutrition to create a holistic approach to well-being.

With years of experience as a chef, Juanita has honed her skills in crafting not only delectable meals but also dishes that prioritize health without compromising on flavor. Her culinary creations are a testament to the belief that nutritious food can be both a source of nourishment and a celebration of taste.

As an accomplished nutritionist and dietitian, Juanita goes beyond the realm of recipes, weaving together the intricate dance of nutrients and their impact on overall health. Her commitment to promoting wellness extends beyond the pages of cookbooks, resonating in every piece of advice she shares with her audience.

Married and blessed with a beautiful family, Juanita understands the importance of fostering a lifestyle that caters to the needs of both adults and children. Her family-friendly approach to healthy living is reflected not only in her recipes but also in the way she encourages households to embrace wellness as a shared journey.

Juanita's unique perspective on the symbiosis of culinary art and nutritional science makes her a sought-after authority in the realm of healthy living. Her work has inspired countless individuals to reevaluate their relationship with food, transforming meals into moments of nourishment, joy, and familial connection.

When she's not in the kitchen or counseling clients, Juanita revels in the simple pleasures of family life. Her dedication to her own family's health echoes in the heartfelt advice and delicious recipes she shares with readers.

Join Juanita Scott on a journey to a revitalized, healthier you. Through her books, consultations, and culinary creations, she invites you to savor the richness of life and health, one mindful bite at a time.

TABLE OF CONTENTS

INTRODUCTION

In a world inundated with dietary trends and nutritional advice, it's easy to overlook the silent heroes within us—the kidneys. These unassuming bean-shaped organs play a vital role in maintaining the delicate balance of our internal environment. As you embark on this culinary journey with the Renal Diet Cookbook For Beginners 2024, consider this a warm welcome, a guide through the maze of kidney health, and an assurance that you've chosen the right companion for your wellness voyage.

The kidneys, often underestimated in their significance, are the unsung champions of our bodies. Filtering blood, removing waste products, regulating fluid balance, and fine-tuning essential minerals—these are just a few tasks that define their role. Yet, we seldom pause to appreciate the intricacies of this silent symphony within us. Your decision to explore a renal diet is not merely a dietary choice; it's a conscious effort to support and nurture these remarkable organs.

Now, let's dispel any apprehensions you might have about delving into the intricacies of the renal diet. The Renal Diet Cookbook For Beginners 2024 is not just a compilation of recipes; it's a comprehensive guide designed with your journey in mind. Here, you'll find a blend of nourishing dishes, practical tips, and an empowering narrative that transcends the limitations often associated with dietary restrictions.

The journey to understanding renal health begins with acknowledging the importance of the kidneys in our overall well-being. By choosing this cookbook, you've signaled your intent to prioritize your health, and that's a commendable step. So, let's explore the fascinating world of the renal diet and uncover the secrets to not only maintaining but enhancing your kidney health.

First, I need you to picture this: two small, bean-shaped organs, each about the size of a fist, quietly filtering around 120 to 150 quarts of blood daily. They process waste products, excess fluids, and electrolytes, ensuring our bodies maintain the delicate balance required for optimal functioning. While their impact is profound, their presence often goes unnoticed until a health challenge surfaces.

Your kidneys are the unsung heroes that tirelessly contribute to the stability of your internal environment. The decision to delve into the world of renal diets is an acknowledgment of their significance and a commitment to supporting their vital functions. As we explore the intricacies of the renal diet, keep in mind that each recipe and guideline is a step towards honoring and preserving the well-being of these remarkable organs.

Now, let's transition to the heart of our exploration—an inspiring narrative that encapsulates the essence of the renal diet. Imagine a world where a cookbook is not merely a collection of recipes but a transformative guide, a companion on a journey of self-discovery and empowerment.

Meet Alex, a beacon of resilience and courage who encountered an unexpected twist in the narrative of their life—the discovery of kidney disease. Faced with this unforeseen challenge, Alex embarked on a profound journey of self-discovery and health exploration, marked not only by dietary adjustments but also by a fundamental shift in perspective.

The revelation of kidney disease was a turning point, a moment that could have been shrouded in despair. Yet, for Alex, it became a catalyst for transformation. Rather than succumbing to fear, Alex chose empowerment. The renal diet, initially perceived as a set of restrictions, emerged as a powerful ally—a pathway to rejuvenation and holistic well-being.

Alex's journey resonates with the experiences of many who, like Alex, found themselves navigating the uncharted waters of kidney health. It's a narrative of culinary innovation, where every recipe becomes an opportunity to explore and create flavors within the confines of kidney-friendly cuisine. The resilience displayed in the face of challenges mirrors the strength that countless individuals discover when confronted with unexpected health conditions.

The story of Alex underscores the capacity of the renal diet to be more than just a regimen—it becomes a lifestyle. It's a journey marked by creativity in the kitchen, a testament to the unwavering spirit that arises in the pursuit of well-being. Through Alex's experience, we glimpse the discovery of a new world of flavors within the realm of renal-friendly cuisine, proving that a diagnosis can be the beginning of a transformative and flavorful chapter in one's life.

THE ESSENCE OF THE RENAL DIET COOKBOOK

As we delve into the Renal Diet Cookbook For Beginners 2024, consider it a guide that transcends the conventional boundaries of dietary restrictions. It's a celebration of flavors, a symphony of nutrients, and a testament to the idea that delicious meals can coexist with kidney health. Now, let me explain what each chapter stands for:

The initial steps into the renal diet may feel like navigating uncharted waters but fear not. The first few chapters take you through the Basics of Renal Nutrition. Here, we unravel the fundamentals—understanding the role of nutrition in kidney health, the overarching principles of the renal diet, and the importance of tailoring dietary plans to individual needs.

Next, we delve into the core elements—protein, sodium, phosphorus, and potassium. Uncover the delicate balance required to support kidney function without overburdening these vital organs. Learn to make informed choices and discover the nuances of nutrient management on this culinary expedition.

"Getting Started with Renal Diet" is not just a chapter; it's your initiation into practical aspects. Discover kidney-friendly foods, master the art of grocery shopping for renal diets, and gain valuable insights into meal planning. This is the foundation upon which we build your culinary journey.

The heart of the cookbook lies in Chapter 4—"Delicious and Kidney-Friendly Recipes." Here, culinary creativity meets renal health. Explore over 100 breakfast ideas, lunch and dinner options, snacks, desserts, beverages, vegetarian recipes, fish, and seafood—all tailored to tantalize your taste buds while respecting the constraints of a renal diet.

"Cooking Techniques for Renal Diets" is not just about preparing meals; it's an art form. Discover healthy cooking methods, learn the magic of flavoring without excess sodium, and explore smart substitutions that elevate your culinary creations.

Life is dynamic, and so is your health. In "Special Considerations for Different Stages of Kidney Disease," we address the evolving needs of your body. From early stages to advanced conditions and the transition to dialysis, this chapter offers tailored guidance for each phase of your journey.

The journey to optimal health is not confined to the plate. In "Lifestyle and Behavioral Strategies," we delve into hydration, physical activity, stress management, and the critical role of sleep. Embrace a holistic approach to well-being that extends beyond dietary considerations.

"Dining Out and Socializing" is not an afterthought—it's an essential aspect of your life. Navigate restaurant menus, revel in the joy of social gatherings, and discover how to travel while adhering to your renal diet. Your culinary adventure extends beyond your kitchen walls.

As we approach the conclusion, explore "Frequently Asked Questions (FAQs)." Here, we address common concerns, debunk misconceptions, and provide expert answers to your queries. It's a reservoir of knowledge to accompany you on your ongoing journey.

In the concluding chapter, celebrate your progress and draw inspiration from success stories. This is not just an ending but a new beginning—a continuation of your journey towards optimal kidney health.

The appendix is not an afterthought; it's your toolkit for success. Access additional resources, explore useful websites and apps, and refer to the glossary for clarification. Measurement conversion charts make every recipe accessible and adaptable to your needs.

In wrapping up this introduction, let me extend my gratitude for choosing the Renal Diet Cookbook For Beginners 2024 as your guide. This is not just a cookbook; it's a companion on your culinary odyssey. May every page, every recipe, and every word empower you to savor the flavors of life while nurturing the silent heroes within—your kidneys.

As we embark on this culinary adventure together, let this introduction serve as a reminder that you are not alone. The Renal Diet Cookbook For Beginners 2024 is more than a collection of recipes; it's a resource, a companion, and a source of empowerment. With each turn of the page, may you find inspiration, guidance, amazing bonuses, and flavors that will nourish not only your body but also your spirit.

Now, let's transition from this introduction into the first chapter, where I'll unravel the basics of kidney health.

CHAPTER 1

UNDERSTANDING THE BASICS OF KIDNEY HEALTH

Kidney illness is projected to impact 31 million people in the United States alone, and one in every ten people worldwide has some sort of kidney disease. Kidney disease, often known as renal disease, is a broad term for kidney diseases that impair function. Chronic kidney disease (CKD) develops when the kidneys lose their ability to filter toxins and waste products from the blood and execute their jobs properly. This might happen suddenly or gradually. Chronic kidney disease (CKD) is divided into five stages.

Every day, our two kidneys filter approximately 120 to 150 quarts of blood to generate approximately 1 to 2 quarts of urine, which is made up of wastes and surplus fluid. Healthy kidneys regulate blood pressure, eliminate waste and water, tell your body to produce red blood cells and help children grow.

In addition to the many stages of chronic kidney disease, or CKD (described below), there are various forms of kidney disease, each with its own set of causes and therapies. The National Kidney Institute (NKI) and this website give in-depth information regarding the disorders that cause Nephrotic Syndrome (NS) and Focal Segmental Glomerulosclerosis (FSGS).

FIVE STAGES OF KIDNEY DISEASE

The National Renal Foundation (NKF) developed a guideline to assist clinicians in determining the severity of renal disease. The NKF classified kidney disease into five stages. Knowing what stage of kidney disease, a person is in allows healthcare providers to deliver the best care possible because each stage demands a different therapy.

To comprehend each level, we must first comprehend how kidney function is assessed. The Glomerular Filtration Rate (GFR) is the most widely used indicator of kidney function. Kidney function is determined by how well your kidneys clear your blood. A blood test to determine the quantity of creatinine in the blood, or serum creatinine, is the most common method of determining GFR. Creatinine levels rise when renal function diminishes.

GFR is calculated using an equation. In addition to serum creatinine, other variables such as age, race, and gender are considered. Weight, blood urea nitrogen (BUN), and serum albumin are all possible additions.

STAGES	KIDNEY FUNCTION/GFR DESCRIPTION
Stage 1	> 90% Normal to High Functions
Stage 2	60-89% Mildly Decreased Functions
Stage 3	30-59% Mild to Moderately Decreased Functions
Stage 4	15-29% Severely Decreased Functions
Stage 5	< 15% Kidney Failure

The five stages of kidney disease, or CKD, are given below, along with the GFR for each stage:

Stage 1 with normal or high GFR (GFR > 90 mL/min)

Stage 2 Mild CKD (GFR = 60-89 mL/min)

Stage 3A Moderate CKD (GFR = 45-59 mL/min)

Stage 3B Moderate CKD (GFR = 30-44 mL/min)

Stage 4 Severe CKD (GFR = 15-29 mL/min)

Stage 5 End Stage CKD (GFR <15 mL/min)

YOUR KIDNEYS & HOW THEY FUNCTION

The kidneys are two bean-shaped organs about the size of your fist. They are located right below the rib cage on each side of your spine. A healthy kidney filters around half a cup of blood each minute, removing wastes and extra water to create urine. Urine travels from the kidneys to the bladder via two thin muscle tubes called ureters, one on each side of the bladder. Urine is stored in your bladder. The urinary tract includes your kidneys, ureters, and bladder.

THE URINARY TRACT

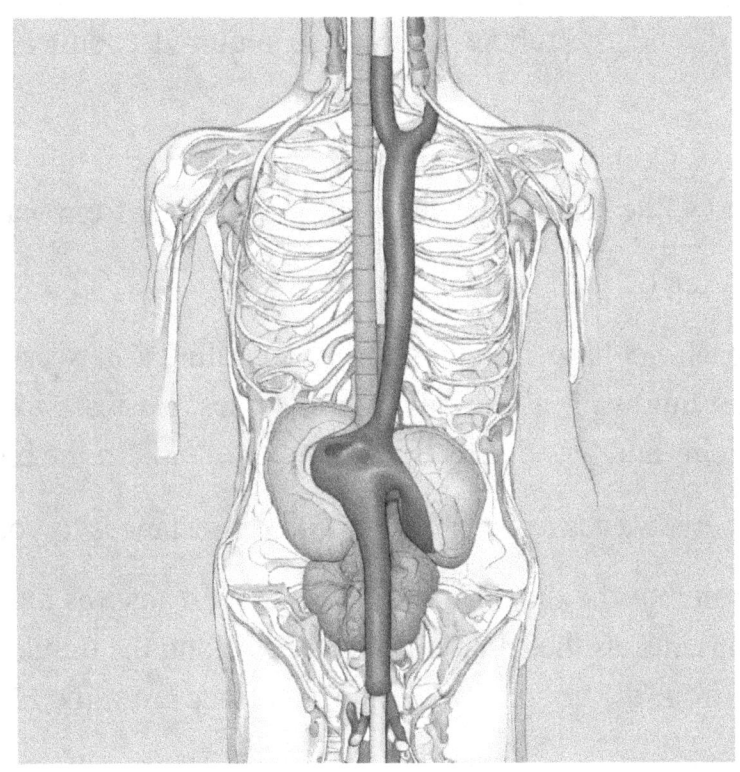

WHAT MAKES THE KIDNEYS SO IMPORTANT?

Your body's kidneys are in charge of eliminating waste and extra fluid. In addition to eliminating acid produced by your body's cells, your kidneys also maintain a normal level of water, salts, and minerals in your blood, including potassium, phosphorus, sodium, and calcium.

- Nerves, muscles, and other tissues in your body may not function normally if this equilibrium is not maintained.
- Your kidneys also produce hormones that aid with digestion.
- keep your blood pressure under control
- red blood cell production
- keep your bones healthy and strong

HOW DO MY KIDNEYS FUNCTION?

Each of your kidneys is made up of about a million filtering units called nephrons. Each nephron has a filter called the glomerulus as well as a tubule. The nephrons filter your blood in two steps:

the glomerulus filters it, and the tubule returns the required chemicals to your blood while removing wastes.

"Each nephron contains a glomerulus that filters your blood and a tubule that restores required substances to your blood while removing waste. Urine is formed from waste and excess water."

- Your blood is filtered by the glomerulus.

As blood rushes into each nephron, it enters the glomerulus, a network of microscopic blood arteries. The glomerulus' thin walls allow smaller molecules, wastes, and fluid—mostly water—to enter the tubule. Proteins and blood cells, for example, remain in the blood vessels.

- The tubule transports wastes and restores required substances to your blood

A blood artery runs parallel to the tubule. The blood vessel reabsorbs almost all of the water, as well as minerals and nutrients, as the filtered fluid passes along the tubule. The tubule aids in the removal of excess acid from the circulation. Urine is formed from the leftover fluid and wastes in the tubule.

HOW DO THE BLOOD VESSELS IN MY KIDNEYS FUNCTION?

The renal artery allows blood to enter your kidney. This huge blood channel divides into smaller blood vessels until the blood reaches the nephrons. Your blood is filtered in the nephron by the microscopic blood vessels of the glomeruli before exiting your kidney via the renal vein.

Your blood passes through your kidneys several times per day. Your kidneys filter around 150 quarts of blood per day. The tubules return the majority of the water and other chemicals that filter through your glomeruli to your blood. Only 1 to 2 quarts are converted to urine. Children produce less pee than adults, and the amount they produce varies with age.

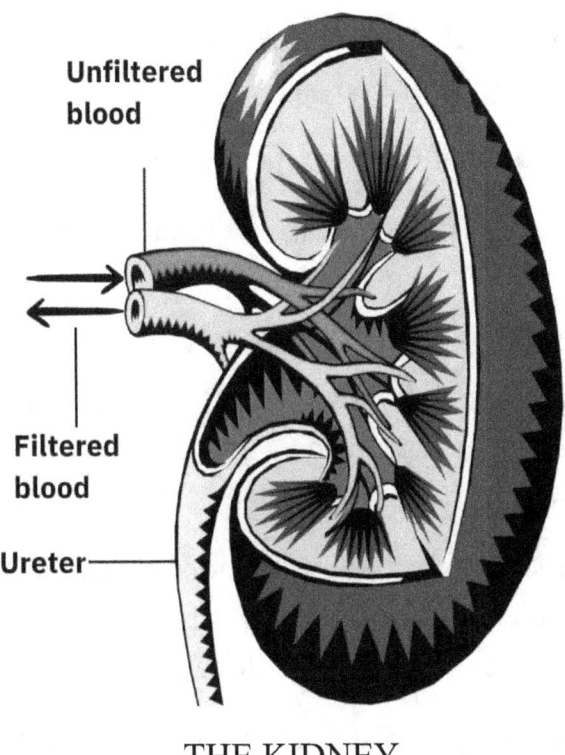

Unfiltered blood

Filtered blood

Ureter

THE KIDNEY

COMMON CAUSES OF KIDNEY DISEASE

Acute kidney disease causes: Acute kidney damage or acute renal failure occurs when your kidneys suddenly cease working. The primary causes are as follows:

- Inadequate blood flow to the kidneys
- Direct kidney injury
- The kidneys were clogged with urine.

These things can occur if you:

- Have a catastrophic injury that results in blood loss, such as getting in a car accident
- Are you dehydrated, or is your muscle tissue deteriorating, releasing an excessive amount of kidney-toxic protein into your bloodstream?
- You are in shock because you have a serious infection known as sepsis.
- Have an enlarged prostate or kidney stones that are preventing urine flow?
- Take some medicines or are exposed to specific poisons that cause direct kidney damage
- Have pregnancy issues such as eclampsia and preeclampsia

- An acute kidney injury can also be caused by autoimmune illnesses, which occur when your immune system attacks your body.

Acute kidney damage is common in those who have severe heart or liver failure.

Chronic kidney disease causes: Chronic renal disease is caused by your kidneys failing to function properly for more than three months. You may not have any symptoms in the early stages, but that is when treatment is easiest.

The most common causes are diabetes (types 1 and 2) and excessive blood pressure. High blood sugar levels might injure your kidneys over time. High blood pressure also causes damage to your blood vessels, especially those leading to your kidneys.

Birth defects can cause urinary tract obstruction or kidney damage. One of the most frequent is a type of valve between the bladder and the urethra. A urologist can frequently perform surgery to correct these issues, which may be discovered while the baby is still in the womb.

Toxins and medicines, such as lead poisoning, long-term use of certain pharmaceuticals, such as NSAIDs (nonsteroidal anti-inflammatory drugs) like ibuprofen and naproxen, and IV street drugs, can irreversibly harm your kidneys. So may prolonged exposure to some substances.

Now, let's move on to the importance of nutrition in your kidney health

THE ROLE OF NUTRITION IN KIDNEY HEALTH

Kidneys are in charge of filtering waste and toxins from our systems and excreting them through urine. They also assist your body in maintaining a healthy balance of nutrients and minerals. As a result, the foods you consume have a direct impact on your kidney health and function. The appropriate nutritious foods can make their work simpler, while others can harm your kidney health. Poor diet is a primary cause of kidney impairment because it can generate high amounts of pollutants in the blood that the kidneys cannot filter out.

A balanced diet also aids in the management of excessive blood sugar and hypertension, two of the primary causes of chronic kidney disease. These disorders damage the blood arteries in the kidney, making it more difficult to filter your blood. Controlling these illnesses and maintaining a healthy weight are critical for kidney health.

SODIUM AND KIDNEY HEALTHY

Consuming too much sodium can be harmful to your kidneys since it raises blood pressure and makes it more difficult for your kidneys to filter waste from your body. As a result, it's critical to keep your daily sodium intake to no more than 2,300 mg, or roughly 1 teaspoon of table salt. This includes avoiding processed and packaged foods and choosing low-sodium alternatives whenever available.

PROTEIN AND KIDNEY HEALTH

Protein is an essential component of a healthy diet. However, if your kidneys aren't functioning properly, eating too much protein can strain them. Because protein degrades into waste, it must be filtered through the kidneys. Protein sources such as lean meats, eggs, beans, and nuts are recommended by experts, as is portion control.

POTASSIUM AND PHOSPHORUS

Phosphorus and potassium are key minerals that help with a range of crucial processes, such as bone strength and heart rate regulation. People with impaired kidney function are at risk of having abnormal levels of these minerals in their blood, which can lead to a variety of health issues. If you have chronic renal disease or another kidney problem, your doctor may advise you to reduce or increase your consumption of certain minerals-rich foods. Phosphorus can be found in processed meals, dark-colored liquids, and animal protein; potassium can be found in fruits, vegetables, and dairy.

FLUIDS AND KIDNEY HEALTH

It's also critical to stay hydrated when trying to keep your kidneys healthy. Drinking sufficient fluids aids in the removal of toxins from the body, allowing your kidneys to operate correctly. However, some fluids, such as alcohol and caffeinated beverages like coffee or soda, can be harmful if consumed in excess. As a result, drink largely water throughout the day and minimize other beverages if possible.

A nutritious diet is essential for optimum kidney health. However, eating healthy isn't always easy, especially if you have diabetes or chronic renal disease. Our specialty programs help make being healthy a bit easier by bringing your supplies straight to your house, from quality testing materials to intermittent catheters.

In recognizing that maintaining a nutritious diet is crucial for optimal kidney health, we acknowledge that the journey to well-being may present its challenges. Especially if you are grappling with diabetes or chronic renal disease, the path to health can seem daunting. Nevertheless, your commitment extends beyond the pages of this cookbook.

This book is designed to not only provide valuable insights and recipes but also to make the health journey more accessible. I understand the unique needs of those navigating chronic renal disease, and my mission is to support you every step of the way. Given that, let's get into Navigating the Renal Pantry, where we will be guiding you through the general list of groceries you will need for most of the recipes in the cookbook, delicious substitutions for your favorite recipes, and foods you'll need to omit. Without further ado, let's dive in.

CHAPTER 2

FOODS TO FAVOR AND FOODS TO AVOID WHEN SHOPPING

GROCERY SHOPPING LIST FOR RENAL DIETS

Note: This is a general grocery shopping list for all foods in this cookbook. Feel free to choose which food items you will need for each recipe.

MEAT/PROTEIN FOODS

- Beef
- Chicken®
- Egg Substitute (Egg Beaters®, Scramblers®)
- Eggs
- Fish
- Lamb
- Pork (chops, roast)
- Shellfish
- Tofu
- Tuna (canned)
- Turkey
- Veal
- Wild Game
- Fruits

VEGETABLES

(Serving size= ½ cup, no added salt)

- Alfalfa Sprouts
- Arugula
- Asparagus
- Bean Sprouts
- Beets (canned)
- Cabbage (green, red)
- Carrots
- Cauliflower
- Celery
- Chayote
- Chili Peppers
- Chives
- Coleslaw
- Corn
- Cucumber
- Eggplant
- Endive
- Garlic
- Ginger Root
- Green Beans
- Hominy
- Jalapenos (fresh)
- Kale
- Leeks
- Lettuce
- Mixed Vegetables
- Mushrooms
- Onions
- Parsley
- Peas (English)
- Pimentos
- Radicchio
- Radishes

- Seaweed Kelp
- Spaghetti Squash
- Summer squash (scallop, crookneck, straight neck, zucchini)
- Sweet Peppers
- Tomatillos
- Turnips
- Turnip Greens
- Water Chestnuts
- Watercress
- Yam Bean (jicama), cooked

BREADS/CEREALS/GRAINS

- Bagels (plain, blueberry, egg, raisin)
- Bread (white, French Italian, rye, soft wheat)
- Bread sticks (plain)
- Cereals, dry, low-salt (Corn Pops®, Cocoa Puffs®, Sugar Smacks®, Fruity Pebbles®, Puffed Wheat®, Puffed Rice®)
- Cereals, cooked (Cream of Rice or Wheat®, Farina®, Malt-o-Meal®)
- Couscous
- Crackers (unsalted)
- Dinner Rolls or Hard Rolls
- English Muffins
- Grits
- Hamburger/Hotdog Bun
- Macaroni
- Melba Toast
- Noodles
- Oyster Crackers
- Pita Bread
- Popcorn (unsalted)
- Pretzels (unsalted)
- Rice (brown, white)
- Rice Cakes
- Spaghetti
- Tortillas

DAIRY/DAIRY SUBSTITUTES

- Non-Dairy Creams
- Non-Dairy Frozen Dessert Topping (Cool Whip®)
- Non-Dairy Frozen Dessert (Mocha Mix®)
- Rice Milk (unfortified)

FRUITS

(Serving size= 1 medium-size fruit or ½ cup canned, no added sugar)

- Apple Juice
- Apples
- Applesauce
- Apricot Nectar
- Apricots (canned)
- Blackberries
- Cherries
- Cranberries
- Cranberry Juice
- Cranberry Sauce
- Figs (fresh)
- Fruit Cocktail
- Grapefruit
- Grape Juice
- Grapes
- Lemon
- Lemon Juice
- Lime
- Lime Juice
- Loganberries
- Lychees
- Peach (canned)
- Peach Nectar
- Pear Nectar
- Pears (canned)
- Pineapple
- Plums
- Raspberries
- Strawberries
- Tangerines

BEVERAGES

(Keep in mind your fluid restriction) (Diabetics- use Caution for sugar intake)

(Regular or Diet)

- 7-Up
- Cherry 7-Up®
- Cream Soda
- Ginger Ale
- Grape Soda
- Lemon-Lime Soda
- Mellow Yellow®
- Mountain Dew®
- Orange Soda
- Root Beer
- Slice®
- Sprite®
- Coffee
- Fruit Punch
- Hi-C® (cherry, grape)
- Horchata
- Juices (apple, cranberry, grape)
- Kool-Aid®
- Lemonade
- Limeade
- Mineral Water
- Nectars (apricot, peach, pear, ½ cup serving)
- Non-Dairy Creamers (Coffee Rich, Mocha Mix®, etc.)
- Sunny Delight®
- Tea

FATS

- Butter
- Cream Cheese
- Margarine
- Mayonnaise
- Miracle Whip®
- Non-Dairy Creamers
- Salad Dressings

- Sour Cream
- Vegetable Oils (preferably canola or olive oil)

SEASONINGS AND SPICES

- Allspice
- Basil
- Bay Leaf
- Caraway Seed
- Chives
- Cilantro
- Cinnamon
- Cloves
- Cumin
- Curry
- Dill
- Extracts (almond, lemon lime, maple, orange, peppermint, vanilla, walnut)
- Fennel
- Garlic Powder
- Ginger
- Horseradish (root)
- Lemon Juice
- Mrs. Dash®
- Nutmeg
- Onion Powder or Flakes
- Oregano
- Paprika
- Parsley or Parsley Flakes
- Pepper (ground)
- Pimentos
- Poppy Seed
- Rosemary
- Saccharin
- Saffron
- Sage
- Savory
- Sesame Seeds
- Tarragon
- Thyme
- Turmeric
- Vinegar

DESSERTS/SNACKS/SWEETS

(Diabetics - use caution)

- Animal Crackers
- Cake (angel food, butter, lemon, pound, spice, strawberry, white, yellow)
- Candy Corn
- Chewing Gum
- Cinnamon Drops
- Cookies (ginger snaps, shortbread, sugar, vanilla wafers)
- Corn Cakes
- Cotton Candy
- Doughnuts
- Fruit Ice
- Graham Crackers
- Gumdrops
- Gummy Bears®
- Hard Candy
- Hot Tamale® Candy
- Jell-O®
- Jelly Beans
- Jolly Ranchers®

16

- Lifesavers®
- Lollipops
- Marshmallows

- Newtons® (fig, strawberry, apple, blueberry)

- Pie (apple, berry, cherry lemon, peach)

OTHERS

(Diabetics – use with caution)

- Apple Butter
- Corn Syrup
- Honey
- Jam

- Jelly
- Maple Syrup
- Marmalade
- Powdered Sugar

- Sugar, brown or white

SUBSTITUTIONS FOR YOUR FAVORITE RECIPES

You can incorporate into your meal plan your favorite recipes from various sources. But it's crucial to leave out or swap out any substances that are bad for your health.

The following foods should be avoided, along with suggestions for alternatives:

Foods to Avoid	Substitution
Bouillon cubes	Homemade stock from cooked chicken or beef
Cakes mix	Homemade cakes
Garlic salt	Fresh or powdered garlic
Instant gravy/sauce mix	Thicken pan dripping with flour or cornstarch
Instant rice and cereals	Long cooking rice and cereals (5 minutes or more)
Onion salt	Fresh or powdered onion
Salt	Spices and herbs

Self-rising cornmeal	Plain cornmeal plus baking powder
Self-rising flour (1 cup)	All purpose flour (1 cup) plus baking powder (1 ½ tablespoon)
Worcestershire or soy sauce (1 teaspoon)	Liquid smoke (1 teaspoon)

LIST OF FOODS TO OMIT

These foods should be omitted from your recipes unless otherwise specified by your Dietitian:

- Apricots
- Baking Soda
- Bananas
- Black-Eyed Peas
- Bouillon Cubes
- Cheese
- Coconut
- Cream Soups
- Cream Style Corn
- Dates
- Dill Pickles

- Instant Mixes
- Instant Rice
- Lima Beans
- Mango
- Melons
- Monosodium Glutamate (MSG)
- Nuts
- Oranges
- Orange Juice
- Potatoes

- Prunes
- Raisins
- Salt
- Sweet Relish Pickles
- Tomatoes
- Tomato Juice
- Tomato Sauce
- Tomato Paste
- Tomato Soup
- Water Chestnuts

HOW TO READ LABELS: A QUICK GUIDE

Serving Size –

Always look here first.

Sodium Goal:

2000 mg a day

600 mg a meal

100 - 200 mg a snack

Sodium –

Always look at the "mg" and NOT the "%"

Ingredient List –

Look for *Phosphorus* or words with "phos" in them.

Phosphoric Acid

Hexametaphosphate

Dicalcium Phosphate

Monocalcium Phosphate

Tricalcium Phosphate

Sodium Phosphate

Stay away from added phosphorus! It adds up to 1000mg phosphorus per day.

Nutrition Facts

Serving Size 2 Tortillas (51g)

Serving per container 6

Amount Per Serving

Calories 110   Calories from Fat 10

	% Daily Value*
Total Fat 1g	2%
Saturated Fat 0g	0%
Trans Fat 0g	0%
Cholesterol 0mg	0%
Sodium 30mg	1%
Total Carbohydrate 22g	7%
Dietary Fiber 2g	9%
Sugar 0g	
Protein 2g	

Vitamin A 0%	*	Vitamin C 0%	
Calcium 2%	*	Iron 4%	

*Percentage Daily Values are based on a 2000 calorie diet. Your daily values may be higher or lower depending on your calorie needs:

Calories per gram:

Fat 9 * Carbohydrate 4 * Protein 4

Ingredients: Cellulose Gum, Ground Corn treated with Lime, Water, Propionic Acid (to preserve freshness), Benzoic Acid (to preserve freshness), Phosphoric Acid (preservative), Dextrose, Guar Gum, Amylase.

If your food has the Daily Value listed for phosphorus, use this guide:

0% - 5% Daily Value – Low Phosphorus (0-50 mg)

5% - 15% Daily Value – Medium Phosphorus (51-150 mg)

Over 15% Daily Value – High Phosphorus (151 mg or higher)

Potassium – listing is not required.

No listing does **NOT** mean no Potassium

CHAPTER 3

ESSENTIAL NUTRIENTS IN RENAL DIETS

Eating healthily is an essential aspect of your treatment and can make you feel better. A fresh diet is a vital aspect of your treatment plan. Not only will it make you feel better, but it may also help you prevent renal disease consequences such as fluid overload, high blood potassium, bone disease, and weight loss.

Because each person is unique and has distinct needs, the following dietary recommendations should be offered based on a variety of circumstances and after consulting with your renal dietician. These considerations include the stage of your kidney illness, the type of treatment you are receiving, test results, and the presence of any other medical disorders.

Kidney function is necessary for eliminating waste from the food you consume. In addition to salt, potassium, and phosphate, the kidneys emit urea, a food protein. These chemicals can accumulate in the body if renal function is hindered. A rigorous diet can help reduce this accumulation and its effects.

Now, here are some essential nutrients to be extremely careful of when considering the food you want to eat:

PROTEIN: QUANTITY AND QUALITY

One of the most hotly debated topics in CKD nutritional therapy is protein intake. A high-protein diet, defined as consuming more than 1.2 grams of protein per kilogram of body weight per day (g/kg/day), has been linked to considerable deterioration in kidney function. High protein intake improves renal blood flow and intraglomerular pressure, resulting in a greater GFR and more effective protein-derived nitrogen excretion.

Hyperfiltration caused by high protein consumption has been described in various experimental models and clinical trials. In the long run, glomerular hyperfiltration caused by a high-protein diet may be harmful to the kidney and other organ systems. Several studies have found that long-term exposure to a high-protein diet can result in kidney injury and progressive renal failure.

The Nurses' Health Study examined the effects of protein intake on estimated GFR based on serum creatinine (eGFRcr) decline in 1,624 women over an 11-year period. The findings revealed that high protein intake was linked with a decrease in eGFRcr in those with impaired kidney function (eGFRcr of 55 to 80 mL/min/1.73 m2) but not in those with normal kidney function. Jhee et al. found that a high-protein diet caused glomerular hyperfiltration and a rapid deterioration in kidney function in the general population.

A high-protein diet raises the risk of renal hyperfiltration and fast deterioration in kidney function in the general population. While the effects of a high-protein diet on those with normal renal function are debatable, excessive protein intake should be avoided in people with CKD or at risk of developing it. In the United States, average dietary protein intake decreases as CKD develops, and dietary protein intake in CKD was above the target level for CKD patients but somewhat below the recommended level in the general population.

A low-protein diet may improve kidney function by lowering capillary hypertension and glomerular hyperfiltration. While experimental research suggests that protein restriction can improve glomerular sclerosis, reduce proteinuria, and preserve GFR, not all clinical trials have found that low-protein diets are effective in CKD patients.

The Modification of Diet in Renal Disease (MDRD) study, the biggest controlled trial of dietary protein management in CKD patients, found that a low-protein diet did not improve outcomes. These findings should be interpreted with caution because the MDRD trial had significant limitations, including a brief follow-up period and a somewhat low rate of diet adherence. Nonetheless, the majority of controlled trials and meta-analyses point to the benefits of dietary protein restriction. A low-protein diet slowed renal function decline and delayed dialysis beginning in patients with advanced CKD.

Furthermore, dietary protein restriction may help with metabolic dysfunction in CKD. A low-protein diet can help CKD patients with metabolic acidosis. Acid is created during the metabolism of proteins. As kidney function diminishes, acid secretion becomes impaired, resulting in persistent metabolic acidosis. Metabolic acidosis reduces protein synthesis, promotes muscle catabolism, and worsens uremic symptoms.

A study of a supplemented extremely low-protein diet found that reducing dietary protein intake decreased metabolic acidosis in individuals with advanced CKD. Dietary adjustment is critical in the treatment of hyperphosphatemia in CKD patients, as dietary protein, particularly animal protein, is a key source of phosphorus. Dietary protein restriction may help reduce hyperphosphatemia, which leads to better control of CKD-MBD.

Inhibiting the renin-angiotensin-aldosterone system (RAAS) is an important part of CKD care since it reduces glomerular hyperfiltration and delays the course of the disease. The combination of RAAS inhibition and dietary protein restriction is thought to provide additive protective effects against renal disease progression. RAAS inhibition and dietary protein restriction have similar effects on renal arteries, reducing glomerular pressure and fibrosis by inhibiting the transforming growth factor-β pathway.

In addition, a low-protein diet may directly reduce kidney RAAS activation, regardless of kidney hemodynamics. Many studies on the effects of low-protein diets were undertaken before the widespread use of RAAS inhibition, so there is little evidence of the effects of low-protein diets in combination with RAAS inhibition.

Two trials found that a low-protein diet paired with an angiotensin-converting enzyme (ACE) inhibitor resulted in an additional reduction in proteinuria. Protein restriction reduced proteinuria by 33% more than the group treated with only an ACE medication. Although there is little data to support the combination of RAAS inhibitors and dietary protein restriction, a low-protein diet is generally recommended for patients with CKD on RAAS inhibitors.

The primary concerns for low-protein diets in clinical practice are the danger of PEW and adherence to dietary limitations. Several trials examining low-protein diets in CKD patients have found satisfactory safety, with no significant consequences and a modest incidence of PEW and malnutrition. A 30-month clinical research investigating low-protein diets in CKD G4, and G5 patients reported that the majority of patients adhered to the prescribed dietary protein restriction, with only 0.7% developing malnutrition.

Another study found that protein restriction in CKD patients had no effect on body composition or skeletal muscle mass. A diet containing 0.6 to 0.8 g/kg/day protein and adequate energy intake (30 to 35 kcal/kg/day) may meet dietary needs in patients with CKD, especially if half of the protein comes from "high biological value protein" sources that contain the essential amino acids in appropriate ratios and amounts, such as eggs, milk, meat, and fish.

While adherence to dietary protein reduction is difficult to predict, excellent patient-physician communication, instruction on simplified dietary options, and regular dietitian surveillance may help.

Although most worldwide Instructions recommend a low-protein diet for CKD patients, protein requirements differ. For individuals with moderate-to-advanced renal disease (eGFRcr < 45 mL/min/1.73 m2) and significant proteinuria (urinary protein excretion > 0.3 g/day), most Instructions suggest a protein intake of 0.6 to 0.8 g/kg/day or a very-low-protein diet with keto acid analogs. Higher protein intake (1.0 to 1.2 g/kg/day) is indicated for KF patients receiving replacement treatment, as more protein is required to prevent PEW.

Patients with nephrotic syndrome may benefit from a low-protein diet (0.8 g/kg/day plus 1 g/day protein for every 1 g urine protein excretion above 5 g/day), as long as they consume enough calories. Furthermore, the target protein intake should be tailored to each patient's clinical condition and illness severity.

Patients with non-protein uric CKD G1, G2, elderly people with CKD G3b, and patients with slowly developing CKD should follow a protein restriction of 0.8 to 1.0 g/kg per day. Several studies have revealed that the protein source influences the course of renal disease. Red meat consumption is specifically linked to an elevated risk of KF, whereas other protein sources, such as chicken, fish, eggs, or dairy products, have no association with KF risk.

Furthermore, dairy products have been linked to a decreased risk of CKD onset and development. However, there is inadequate data to prescribe certain protein types for people with CKD. It is recommended that people with CKD consume at least half of their protein consumption from sources with "high biological value."

CONTROLLING SODIUM INTAKE

High salt intake has a negative impact on blood pressure, cardiovascular health, renal function, and CKD progression. Dietary salt restriction is strongly advised in CKD patients to regulate fluid retention, lower blood pressure, and reduce cardiovascular risk. A randomized controlled trial found that sodium restriction reduced blood pressure, extracellular fluid volume, and proteinuria in individuals with moderate-to-severe CKD.

Furthermore, sodium restriction increased the positive effects of a low-protein diet and RAAS inhibition by lowering intraglomerular pressure, implying that sodium restriction may reduce proteinuria and slow the course of CKD. However, there is equivocal evidence that dietary salt restriction can decrease the advancement of kidney disease or postpone the need for renal replacement treatment.

A longitudinal investigation demonstrated that dietary sodium intake had no effect on renal disease development, however, another study found that sodium excretion was connected with CKD progression and all-cause mortality in 3,939 patients with CKD. The highest quartile of urinary sodium excretion ($\geq$ 4.5 g/day) was linked with a 54% greater risk of CKD progression and a 45% increase in mortality compared to the lowest quartile (< 2.7 g/day).

Almost all Instructions indicate that adults limit their sodium consumption to 2 to 2.3 g per day. Patients with severe CKD and dialysis should not consume less than 1.5 g of salt per day due to the risk of hyponatremia and unfavorable consequences. Patients with CKD should be advised to avoid processed foods and cook their own meals without salty seasonings.

Although 24-hour urine collection provides the gold standard for quantifying salt intake, it is inconvenient. To assess and monitor dietary salt consumption, employ the urinary sodium excretion rate from spot urine or the sodium frequency meal questionnaire. However, urinary sodium excretion proved ineffective in evaluating the effects of a low-sodium diet in CKD patients. As a result, it is vital to assess patients' dietary salt intake and educate them depending on their individual circumstances.

In short, to limit your sodium intake, you should:

- Avoid table salt and other spices that end with the word "salt".
- Avoid salt replacements (which include potassium).
- Avoid eating salty meats including bacon, ham, sausage, hot dogs, lunch meats, canned meats, and bologna.
- Avoid eating salty snacks like cheese curls, crackers, almonds, and chips.
- Avoid canned soups, freezer meals, and instant noodles.
- Avoid bottled sauces, pickles, olives and MSG.

CONTROLLING YOUR POTASSIUM LEVELS

Potassium, as the primary intracellular cation, regulates intracellular electrophysiology and is essential for vascular and neuromuscular function. Serum potassium levels are tightly controlled, as low potassium is associated with muscular weakness and hypertension, while high potassium can cause cardiac arrhythmia and mortality. As a result, dietary potassium intake and serum potassium levels are of substantial therapeutic importance. However, few research have looked into the effects of dietary changes on serum potassium levels in CKD patients.

Several studies have used urine potassium excretion as a surrogate for dietary potassium consumption to investigate the impact on clinical outcomes. Nonetheless, there is limited evidence to support the assumption that dietary potassium restriction improves the outcomes of CKD patients, and the majority of recommendations are based on opinion. The 2015 American Dietary Instructions Advisory Committee study advises that healthy individuals consume 4,700 mg (121 mmol) of potassium per day.

The National Kidney Foundation Kidney Disease Outcomes Quality Initiative Instructions propose a potassium intake of 2 to 4 g/day (51 to 102 mmol/day) for individuals with CKD G3, G4, but no limitations (> 4 g/day or > 102 mmol/day) for those with earlier stages of CKD. The average dietary potassium intake in Korea was observed to be 88% of the recommended amount in males and 72% in women, with cereals, vegetables, and pork being the most common food sources of potassium.

Aside from kidney function and dietary intake, several other factors influence serum potassium levels, including the use of RAAS and beta-blockers, hydration status, acid-base status, glycemic control, adrenal function, catabolic state, and gastrointestinal problems such as diarrhea, constipation, or bleeding. Because there has been little research into the effects of these factors, a personalized treatment for each patient is recommended.

Previous observational studies have found that a plant-based diet is related to a slower drop in eGFRcr among CKD patients. Consuming more plant-based foods, such as vegetables and grains, rather than animal-based foods, such as red meat, may help prevent or reduce the course of CKD, type 2 diabetes, high blood pressure, and heart disease. Eating less animal-based meals can reduce acid load and put less strain on the kidneys. Furthermore, plant-based foods that are not excessively processed include phytates. Because phytates can bind phosphate, plant-based diets are expected to absorb far less phosphate than highly processed foods.

A potassium-rich diet, such as a plant-based diet, may have limited efficacy in managing serum potassium and phosphate levels in people with kidney disease. Therefore, customized approaches to dietary potassium consumption in patients with CKD should target a normal- to high-potassium diet.

If hyperkalemia is a concern in CKD patients, potassium binders could be utilized to give a more liberalized potassium diet that includes fruits and vegetables. However, no studies have been conducted to determine whether potassium consumption should be changed when taking potassium binders. The most recent Instructions propose that individuals with CKD alter their dietary potassium intake on an individual basis to maintain normal serum potassium levels.

In other words, a renal patient's diet should contain no more than 2000 mg of potassium per day.

Here are some foods that are high in potassium:

- Avocado
- Oranges
- Orange Juice
- Prunes
- Prune Juice
- Tomatoes
- Tomato Juice
- Tomato Sauce

- Tomato Puree
- Honeydew Melon
- Papaya
- Bananas
- Cantaloupe
- Chocolate
- Nuts
- Red Beans

- White Beans
- Lima Beans
- Garbanzo Beans
- Black Beans
- Lentils
- Split peas
- Baked Beans
- Milk

CONTROLLING YOUR PHOSPHORUS LEVELS

Most natural and processed meals contain phosphorus, which is a necessary component for maintaining homeostasis. Phosphorus is required for bone formation and mineralization, as well as the management of energy and acid-base balance. During the early stages of CKD (eGFRcr > 45 mL/min/1.73 m2), patients with CKD often maintain normal blood phosphorus levels by increasing fibroblast growth factor 23 (FGF-23) and parathyroid hormone (PTH) levels, which promote phosphorus excretion. However, when CKD continues, resistance to FGF-23 and PTH can cause high serum phosphate levels, often known as hyperphosphatemia.

Elevated serum phosphorus levels have been linked to increased cardiovascular risk in both CKD patients and the general population. A recent study highlighted the mechanism linked with increased cardiovascular risk in hyperphosphatemia, which can promote left ventricular hypertrophy and arterial stiffness by inducing FGF-23 and vascular calcification [67,68]. Dietary phosphate intake, as evaluated by 24-hour urine phosphate excretion, had no effect on the development of KF or cardiovascular mortality while serum phosphorus levels were normal.

Traditional Instructions recommend that patients with CKD G3-5 and KF on dialysis consume 800 to 1,000 mg of phosphorus per day to keep their serum phosphate levels within normal ranges. It is unclear how to reduce dietary phosphorus in adult individuals with CKD. Furthermore, the type of dietary protein that serves as the principal source of phosphorus influences its amount and bioavailability. Instructions that propose lowering dietary phosphorus intake frequently raise concerns about the risk of limiting protein intake in CKD patients, particularly those on maintenance dialysis. As a result, dietary consults should include information regarding phosphorus-containing protein sources as well as recommendations for cooking phosphate-rich foods to achieve minimal phosphorus intake without sacrificing nutritional quality. In addition, patient education on hyperphosphatemia therapy, such as adopting a low-phosphate diet and using phosphate binders appropriately, may enhance phosphate control.

Additional plant-based sources of phosphorus may be used in nutritional management because gastrointestinal absorption of plant-based phosphorus (20% to 50%) is lower than that of animal-based diets (40-60%). Furthermore, phosphorus-containing dietary additives in processed and fast foods are of special concern since they include inorganic phosphorus, which is almost completely absorbed in the gut.

Recent Instructions emphasize personalized recommendations based on dietary phosphorus intake to keep serum phosphorus levels within the normal range in individuals with CKD. To lower the pill burden of phosphate binders in patients with advanced CKD, consider restricting the intake of animal-based dietary phosphates and replacing them with plant-derived dietary phosphates.

In other words, take into consideration the following advice to maintain healthy levels of phosphorus:

1. Eat less items high in phosphorus, such as:
- Meats, poultry, dairy products, and fish (one serving should be about 7-8 ounces).
- Milk and other dairy products, such as cheese (one 4-ounce serving is recommended)

2. Steer clear of foods high in phosphorus, such as:
- Garbanzo beans, lime beans, black beans, red beans, black-eyed peas, and white beans.
- Whole, dark, or unprocessed grains
- Doughs for refrigerators, like Pillsbury
- Fruits and vegetables that have been dried

- Chocolate
- Sodas with a dark color

3. Remember to always take your phosphate binders with meals and snacks.
- A calcium supplement or polymer gel prescription known as a phosphate binder will be prescribed by your doctor. Phosphate binder must be taken exactly as directed by your physician. Phosphate binder is often taken with every meal and snack.

4. Typically, the daily allowance of phosphorus in your diet is 1000 mg.

CONTROLLING YOUR FLUID INTAKE

People on dialysis frequently have decreased urine output, thus excess fluid in the body can place unneeded strain on the heart and lungs.

- Individual patients' fluid allowance is determined as 'urine plus 500ml.' The 500 ml includes fluid loss through the skin and lungs.
- Most patients will notice a decrease in urination after starting hemodialysis. Others who create a lot of pee may be able to drink more than others who do not produce any.
- Patients should anticipate gaining some weight between dialysis treatments due to the water content of diets (fruits and vegetables).
- A typical day's meal contains at least 500 ml of fluid (excluding fluids such as water, tea, and so on), hence the daily weight gain is estimated to be between 0.4 and 0.5kg.

Patients should follow these Instructions to regulate their fluid consumption:

- To maintain proper fluid consumption, patients should not exceed their doctor's recommended amount (about 4 cups per day).
- Count all food items that melt at room temperature (Jell-O®, popsicles, and fruit juices).

As we conclude this chapter, you've learned about the complexities of controlling important nutrients during your renal diet journey. You now have a better understanding of how protein, salt, phosphorus, and potassium affect kidney health.

Remember, this chapter is more than just a set of principles; it's a road map for your health. Mastering the art of nutrition regulation not only nourishes your body but also provides you with the tools you need to negotiate the complexity of a renal diet.

Allow this understanding to guide you as you move forward. Every decision you make about managing critical nutrients is a step toward maintaining and improving your kidney health. In the following chapters, we'll look at practical tips, delectable recipes, and insights to make your renal diet journey both enriching and fun.

So, take a minute to reflect on what you've learned, enjoy your accomplishments, and prepare for the culinary adventures ahead. Your dedication to studying and managing critical nutrients demonstrates your proactive approach to well-being.

Here's to your continued success on this journey to optimal kidney health!

CHAPTER 4

BREAKFAST RECIPES

1. FRUIT AND OAT PANCAKES

Cook time: 30 mins   **Yield:** 6 Pancakes

Ingredients

- 4 ounces of fruit cocktail.
- 1 teaspoon of lemon zest.
- Combine 1/2 cup rolled oats, 2 tablespoons heavy cream, and 1/2 cup water.
- One huge egg.
- 1/2 tbsp brown sugar
- ½ teaspoon vanilla.
- 1/2 teaspoon baking powder.
- ½ teaspoon cinnamon.
- ¼ teaspoon nutmeg.
- ¼ cup flour

Instructions

- Add the fruit cocktail to a food processor or blender. Blend until small parts remain but are not completely pureed. If necessary, add 1 or 2 tablespoons of the cream-water mixture to help it combine.
- Mix in the lemon zest and leave aside.
- Let the oats and cream-water combination stand for 1 minute.
- Stir in the egg until thoroughly combined.
- Add the brown sugar and vanilla, and stir well.
- Combine baking powder, cinnamon, nutmeg, and flour. Stir just enough to moisten the dry ingredients.
- Stir in the fruit cocktail and zest mixture until thoroughly combined.
- Heat a small pan on medium-low heat. When hot, spritz with olive oil.
- Pour ¼ cup batter into the pan and spread out slightly.
- Allow to cook for about 2 minutes, or until the edges are dry and the spatula slides beneath the pancake without breaking it.
- Flip and cook for 1 to 2 minutes, or until browned. If the browning occurs too quickly, reduce the heat. Make sure your spatula is thoroughly under the pancake. These are delicate and can break if not properly supported underneath.
- Spray the pan again with olive oil, then continue with the remaining batter.
- Serve two pancakes and top with syrup (if preferred).

Nutritional Facts: Calories 179kcal, Fat 8g, Carbohydrates 25g, Protein 6g, Sodium 107mg, Calcium 82mg, Phosphorus 124mg, Potassium 155mg

2. Bell Pepper and Feta Crustless Quiche

Cook time: 40 mins   **Yield:** 5

Ingredients

- 1 teaspoon olive oil, plus enough for the pie plate.
- 1 tiny sweet onion, diced.
- 1 teaspoon minced garlic.
- One red bell pepper, chopped
- 1 cup homemade rice milk (or unsweetened store-bought)
- 4 eggs
- ¼ cup all-purpose flour
- ¼ cup feta cheese (low sodium).
- 2 teaspoons of fresh basil leaves, chopped
- Black pepper, freshly ground, to taste

Instructions

- Preheat the oven to 400° Fahrenheit.
- Lightly coat a 9-inch pie pan in olive oil.
- In a medium skillet over medium-high heat, heat 1 teaspoon olive oil.
- Sauté the onion and garlic until softened, about 3 minutes.
- Stir in the bell pepper and sauté for about 3 minutes.
- Transfer the vegetables to the prepared pie plate.
- In a medium bowl, combine the rice milk, eggs, and flour.
- Add the feta cheese and basil, and season with black pepper.
- Pour the egg mixture onto the vegetables in the pie plate. Bake for approximately 20 minutes, or until the center is set and the edges are golden brown.
- Serve either hot, warm, or cold.

Nutritional Facts: Calories 162kcal, Fat 6g, Carbohydrates 19g, Protein 8g, Sodium 154mg, Calcium 129mg, Phosphorus 135mg, Potassium 143mg

3. Mexican Brunch Eggs

Cook time: 30 mins   **Yield:** 8

Ingredients

- 1/2 cup diced onion
- 2 garlic cloves, smashed
- Two tablespoons margarine
- 1 1/2 cups frozen corn, thawed
- 1 1/2 tablespoons ground cumin
- 1/8 teaspoon of cayenne pepper.
- Eight eggs, beaten
- 8 slices of toasted bread.

Instructions

- In a large skillet, cook the onion and garlic in margarine until the onion is tender.

- Stir in the corn, cumin, and cayenne until combined.
- Pour in the eggs or egg substitute and simmer on low heat, stirring regularly, until set.
- Arrange the bread triangles on a wide dish.
- Spoon egg mixture onto bread triangles.
- Serve immediately.

Nutritional Facts: Calories 214kcal, Fat 20g, Carbohydrates 13g, Protein 9g, Sodium 147mg, Calcium 86mg, Phosphorus 91mg, Potassium 240mg

4. FRENCH TOAST

Cook time: 10 mins   **Yield:** 1

Ingredients

- 1 teaspoon of butter
- 1 medium-sized egg
- 50 mL of (2 fluid ounces) reduced fat milk
- 1 thick slice from a large loaf of bread
- 1 tablespoon maple syrup

Instructions

- Whisk together the egg and milk.
- Coat the bread with egg and milk mixture.
- In a frying pan, melt the butter over medium heat.
- Add the bread to the pan and cook for 2 to 3 minutes on each side.
- Finish with maple syrup.

Nutritional Facts: Calories 239kcal, Fat 11g, Carbohydrates 30g, Protein 5g, Sodium 0.9g, Phosphate 128mg, Potassium 128mg

5. EGG SANDWICH

Cook time: 15 mins   **Yield:** 1

Ingredients

- Two slices of wheat bread
- 3 medium basil leaves and ½ tbsp olive oil.
- 1 egg
- 1 tablespoon of water.
- Add a pinch of salt and black pepper.
- 1 piece of cheddar cheese.
- 2 slices of medium tomato.

Instructions

- Toast the bread in a dry skillet or toaster. Set aside.
- Remove the basil leaves from their stalks and set them aside.
- Cook in a small skillet over medium heat. Add the olive oil.
- Scramble the eggs with water. Season the eggs with salt and pepper.
- Pour into a skillet. Cook in a single layer, like an omelet. Don't fold in half. Flip and fry the other side.

- Layer the cheese over the warm slice of bread, followed by the egg. Fold the edges under to accommodate the bread's size. Add tomato slices to the eggs, then the basil leaves. Top with the second slice of bread.
- Cut the sandwich in half diagonally. Serve while hot! Enjoy!

Nutritional Facts: Calories 385kcal, Fat 22g, Carbohydrates 30g, Protein 18g, Sodium 630mg, Calcium 252mg Phosphorus 262mg, Potassium 214mg

6. ASPARAGUS & SWISS CHEESE FRITTATA

Cook time: 50 mins   **Yield:** 1

Ingredients

- Three huge eggs.
- 5 egg whites (if boxed, use ¼ cup plus 2 teaspoons).
- 2 tablespoons grated Parmesan cheese with decreased sodium content
- 1 tablespoon of heavy cream.
- 3 ounces Swiss cheese, shredded and divided
- 1/8 teaspoon pepper
- 1 tablespoon of unsalted butter.
- Ingredients: ½ cup chopped shallots, ½-pound asparagus with rough ends removed and sliced into ½-inch pieces (about 4 ounces).

Instructions

- Whisk together the eggs, egg whites, Parmesan, heavy cream, half of the Swiss cheese, and pepper. Set aside.
- Melt the butter in a 12-inch oven-safe nonstick pan over medium heat.
- Add the shallots and simmer for 2 minutes.
- Cook for a further two minutes after adding the asparagus.
- Turn the heat down to the lowest level.
- Give the egg mixture a final whisk before adding it to the pan. Make careful to completely cover the bottom and do not stir.
- Allow to cook for 10 minutes, or until the center is just set.
- While that is cooking, put the broiler to high (500°F).
- When the eggs are cooked, remove from the heat, remove the cover, and sprinkle the remaining half of the Swiss cheese on top.
- Broil for two minutes, or until the cheese has melted.
- Cut into four equal wedges and serve hot.

Nutritional Facts: Calories 241kcal, Fat 16g, Carbohydrates 7g, Protein 18g, Sodium 162mg, Calcium 261mg Phosphorus 257mg, Potassium 323mg

7. BLUEBERRY PEANUT BUTTER OATMEAL

Prep time: 5 mins   **Yield:** 4

Ingredients

- Two cups of traditional oats
- 2 cups unsweetened almond milk
- 2 tablespoons honey
- One tablespoon chia seeds, two tablespoons honey, and two cups of unsweetened almond milk
- One tsp of cinnamon
- Half a cup of peanut butter cereal
- One cup of blueberries

Instructions

- In an airtight jar, combine old fashioned oats, almond milk, honey, chia seeds, and cinnamon.
- Combine and refrigerate for the entire night.
- Spoon a cup of overnight oatmeal into a small bowl when you're ready to eat.
- Add a ¼ cup of fresh blueberries and two spoonfuls of peanut butter granola on top.

Nutritional Facts: Calories 218kcal, Fat 6g, Carbohydrates 39g, Protein 6g, Sodium 13mg, Calcium 83mg Phosphorus 180mg, Potassium 208mg

8. EGG & RICE MUFFINS

Total Cooking time: 27 mins   Yield: 6

Ingredients

- ¾ cup cooked short-grain rice (or ¼ cup cooked plus 2 tablespoons of raw rice)
- Diced pimentos, 1½ ounce (3 teaspoons)
- Two ounces of chopped green chiles (four teaspoons)
- 4 ounces of cheese shreds, split among 3 large eggs
- One-third cup whole milk
- ½ teaspoon of cumin powder
- One-half teaspoon of black pepper

Instructions

- Set oven temperature to 400°F.
- Combine 2 ounces of shredded cheese, pimentos, green chiles, and cooked rice.
- Fill 12-muffin tin with mixture, spooning it in.
- Whisk together the milk and eggs. Add pepper and cumin.
- Transfer mixture to identical muffin pan.
- Dredge remaining cheese onto each of the twelve muffins.
- Bake until hard, 12 to 15 minutes. Allow it cool in the pan for five minutes, then take it out to serve.

Nutritional Facts: Calories 161kcal, Fat 10g, Carbohydrates 19g, Protein 9g, Sodium 162mg, Calcium 166mg Phosphorus 154mg, Potassium 107mg

9. ITALIAN EGGS AND PEPPERS

Cooking time: 30 mins   **Yield:** 3 cups

Ingredients

- One cup of green bell pepper
- half a cup of onions
- one-fourth cup of fresh basil
- Eight big eggs
- 1/4 tsp black pepper
- 1/8 teaspoon of optionally crushed chili flakes

Instructions

- Chop the basil, onion, and bell pepper.
- Cook and sauté onion and green pepper in oil in a big skillet until they are soft.
- Add crushed chile flakes and black pepper after beating eggs until well combined. Add to the skillet along with green peppers and onion.
- Cook on medium heat. Using a spatula, carefully raise the cooked piece as the mixture starts to firm at the bottom and sides to allow the uncooked egg to fall to the bottom. Don't stir all the time.

- Cook for 3 to 5 minutes, or until eggs are thickened all over but still moist. Top with fresh basil and serve hot.

Nutritional Facts: Calories 194kcal, Fat 14g, Carbohydrates 5g, Protein 13g, Sodium 141mg, Calcium 64mg Phosphorus 203mg, Potassium 222mg

10. HOMEMADE MUESLI

Cooking time: 15 mins   **Yield:** 5½

Ingredients

- One cup of dried and coarsely chopped apples
- ½ cup of finely chopped dried apricots
- half a cup of chia seeds
- One-third cup shredded unsweetened coconut
- Half a cup of peeled pumpkin seeds
- ½ cup of cranberries, dried
- 1/4 cup of raisins
- One-half cup rolled oats
- A quarter cup honey

Instructions

- Add the apricots and dried apples to a large mixing bowl.
- Incorporate the oats, chia seeds, coconut, pumpkin seeds, cranberries, and raisins.
- Blend until thoroughly blended.

- When the mixture is just a little lumpy (but not sticky), add the honey and continue to combine.
- Savor it as an independent snack or combine it with normal or non-dairy yogurt, nut milk, or both.

Nutritional Facts: Calories 211kcal, Fat 7g, Carbohydrates 36g, Protein 5g, Sodium 13mg, Calcium 44mg Phosphorus 196mg, Potassium 292mg

- For about 20 minutes, or until the tofu takes on a faint golden-brown color, stir and simmer over low to medium heat. The mixture will lose water through evaporation.
- Warm tofu scrambler is served.

Nutritional Facts: Calories 213kcal, Fat 13g, Carbohydrates 10g, Protein 18g, Sodium 24mg, Calcium 274mg Phosphorus 242mg, Potassium 467mg

11. SPICY TOFU SCRAMBLER

Cooking time: 30 mins   **Yield:** 2

Ingredients

- One tsp olive oil
- ¼ cup chopped red bell pepper
- ¼ cup chopped green bell pepper
- One cup firm tofu with a calcium content of no more than 10%
- One tsp powdered onion
- One-half teaspoon of powdered garlic
- one minced garlic clove
- One-half teaspoon of turmeric

Instructions

- Heat olive oil in a medium-sized nonstick skillet and sauté the garlic and both bell peppers.
- After draining and rinsing, break the tofu into the skillet. Stir in the remaining components.

12. COTTAGE CHEESE PANCAKES

Cooking time: 30 mins   **Yield:** Two 4" Pancakes

Ingredients

- One cup cottage cheese
- Four sizable eggs, lightly whisked
- Half a cup of white all-purpose flour
- Six teaspoons of melted unsalted butter
- Three cups of freshly cut strawberries

Instructions

- Mix the cottage cheese, melted butter, flour, and lightly beaten eggs in a medium-sized bowl.
- Apply butter or non-stick cooking spray on the griddle or frying pan.

- Place a frying pan or griddle over medium-high heat. To make pancakes, ladle about 1/4 cup of batter onto the griddle (about 4" in diameter).
- Cook pancakes for two to three minutes, or until lightly browned on the undersides, then flip and brown on the other side.
- Flip the pancakes over onto a preheated plate.
- Using the leftover batter, keep making pancakes.
- Place half a cup of cut strawberries on top of each pancake serving.

Nutritional Facts: Calories 253kcal, Fat 17g, Carbohydrates 21g, Protein 11g, Sodium 173mg, Calcium 64mg Phosphorus 159mg, Potassium 217mg

13. SPICY CORNBREAD

Cooking time: 30 mins   **Yield**: 8

Ingredients

- One cup of white all-purpose flour
- One cup of basic cornmeal
- One tablespoon each of sugar and baking powder
- One tsp of chili powder
- 1/4 tsp black pepper
- One cup of unenriched rice milk
- One egg
- One white egg

- Two tsp of canola oil
- Half a cup of finely chopped scallions
- 1/4 cup finely shredded carrots
- one minced clove of garlic

Instructions

- Set oven temperature to 400°F.
- Mix the flour, cornmeal, sugar, baking powder, chili powder, and pepper in a large bowl. Mix everything together.
- Stir just until moistened after adding rice milk, egg, egg white, and oil to the dry ingredients.
- Stir the garlic, carrots, and scallions gently into the cornmeal mixture.
- Fill an 8-inch-square baking pan with batter after spraying it with nonstick cooking spray.
- Bake until the top begins to turn golden brown, 25 to 30 minutes. In eight 2" x 4" pieces, cut.

Nutritional Facts: Calories 188kcal, Fat 5g, Carbohydrates 31g, Protein 5g, Sodium 155mg, Calcium 84mg Phosphorus 81mg, Potassium 100mg

14. VEGETARIAN SUMMER ROLLS

Cooking time: 30 mins   **Yield:** 4

Ingredients

Peanut Sauce

- 1/4 cup unsalted natural peanut butter
- Two tsp of coconut aminos
- Add at least 2 tablespoons of canned coconut milk to thicken the sauce.
- One tablespoon of lime juice or rice vinegar
- Two tsp melted coconut oil
- one grated garlic clove
- Half a teaspoon of hot Sriracha sauce not required

Summer Rolls

- Cut one medium cucumber into matchsticks, about 3/4 cup.
- Cut 1/4 medium jicama into matchsticks, about 1 cup
- One cup of shredded red cabbage
- Eight tiny, halved green lettuce leaves
- 1/4 cup finely chopped mint, cilantro, or basil
- Dice one avocado into eight thin pieces.
- One tsp toasted sesame seeds eight round, 8 to 9-inch rice cakes

Instructions

- Combine all the ingredients in a basin and whisk to blend them into a peanut sauce. As needed, adjust the consistency and seasoning.

- Before assembling your rolls, prepare all of your vegetables.
- Get a small bowl ready, fill it with room temperature water, and wet a plate or cutting board, or any flat surface will do.
- Rice paper can be made softer by soaking it in water for three to five seconds, or as directed on the packaging. Though not floppy, the rice paper should be somewhat pliable and softer than before. As you add the fillings, it will continue to soften quickly.
- The soaked rice paper should be placed on a damp surface. Place your sliced avocado in the center, followed by some sesame seeds, herbs, and a small amount of each vegetable. Take care not to pack rolls too full for wrapping.
- After that, using wet hands, wrap the summer roll by folding the sides inside, folding the bottom side upward, and rolling upward until it is sealed. Continue with the remaining rolls.
- Enjoy right away with peanut sauce on the side.

Nutritional Facts: Calories 325kcal, Fat 17g, Carbohydrates 37g, Protein 9g, Sodium 423mg, Calcium 72mg, Potassium 491mg

Notes

It's possible that you've heard that due to their high phosphorus content, whole grains, beans, and nuts are not the best options for a kidney-friendly diet. Are you wondering why so many of our recipes call for them? Since people only absorb roughly 40% of the phosphorus found in plant foods like beans, nuts, and whole grains, we include them. They therefore suit the majority of people's diets well! Please contact your dietician if you have any queries about including these foods in your diet.

15. STUFFED GREEN PEPPERS

Cooking time: 20 mins   **Yield:** 6

Ingredients

- Three bell peppers, green
- One pound of ground beef
- Two tsp unsalted butter (to be used in two portions)
- 1/4 cup finely chopped onions
- Three tablespoons of mild, chunky, thick salsa
- One tsp Mrs. Dash® herb and onion seasoning
- two cups of boiled rice
- half a cup of water
- Half a cup of moist white breadcrumbs
- One tsp poultry seasoning
- One tsp of paprika

Instructions

- Peel and cut the peppers in half lengthwise. Take out the seeds. For four minutes, parboil.
- Grind the beef and sauté it in a big skillet. Take out the meat and set it aside. Throw away pan drippings.
- Fry one onion in one tsp margarine till it becomes transparent. Place the cooked rice, meat, salsa, and Mrs. Dash® herb spice on top. Mix everything together.
- Place the meat and rice mixture inside the green pepper halves, then press the halves onto a shallow baking dish. Fill the pan with 1/2 cup of water.
- Mix melted butter, chicken spice, and bread crumbs together. Over the stuffed peppers, sprinkle.
- Bake, covered, for 30 minutes at 350 F. Bake uncovered for 5 minutes, or until golden.

Nutritional information: 259 kcal, 12g fat, 20g carbs, 16g protein, 152 mg sodium, 29 mg calcium. Potassium 313 mg and Phosphorus 132 mg

16. GERMAN PANCAKES

Cooking time: 25 mins   **Yield:** 2

Ingredients

- 2/3 cup flour of all purposes
- two tsp sugar

- Four big eggs
- One cup low-fat milk (1%).
- One-fourth teaspoon of vanilla essence

Instructions

- Mix the flour and sugar together in a medium-sized bowl. Whisk the eggs in thoroughly after adding them.
- Mix in the vanilla extract and milk. Until smooth, beat.
- After sprinkling nonstick cooking spray over an 8" or 10" heated nonstick pan, transfer 3 tablespoons of the batter into the skillet. To spread the batter, quickly tilt the pan. Cook for about 45 seconds, or until the pancake's underside is brown; the edges will start to dry up. After flipping, brown the other side of the pancake. Proceed until all of the batter has been used.
- Serve thin pancakes with jam, syrup, or fruit spread after folding or rolling them. If filling is preferred, add 1 to 2 tablespoons of cream cheese or ricotta.

Nutritional Facts: Calories 74kcal, Fat 2g, Carbohydrates 10g, Protein 4g, Sodium 39mg, Calcium 43mg Phosphorus 72mg, Potassium 73mg

17. TOFU SCRAMBLE

Cooking time: 35 mins   **Yield:** 5

Ingredients

- Firm, drained 19 ounces (539 grams) of tofu
- Three tablespoons of flakes of nutritious yeast
- Two tsp Dijon mustard
- Two teaspoons of pasted tahini
- One tablespoon of powdered smoked paprika
- One tablespoon of powdered turmeric
- two tsp water
- Two tsp olive oil
- One small onion (54 grams), diced
- 3 2/3 cup (100 grams) uncooked, washed, and sliced kale
- One little (seventy grams) sliced plum tomato

Instructions

- In a bowl, crumble the drained tofu.
- In a small bowl, mix together nutritional yeast flakes, Dijon mustard, tahini, smoked paprika, turmeric, and water. Mix thoroughly with a whisk. Stir in the crumbled tofu and stir once more.
- In a medium skillet over medium heat, warm the olive oil. Cook the onion for five minutes on low heat after adding it.
- Add the kale and stir for about three minutes, or until the kale wilts.
- To the skillet, add the tofu mixture.

- Cook and stir until the tofu and kale are well combined and cooked, about 5 minutes.
- Split into five equal parts. Garnish each serving on a separate plate with a little sliced tomato.

Nutritional Facts: Calories 239kcal, Fat 2g, Carbohydrates 11.2g, Protein 18g, Sodium 189mg, Calcium 379mg Phosphorus 300mg, Potassium 503mg

18. APPLE FRITTER RINGS

Cooking time: 28 mins   **Yield:** 1

Ingredients

- Four big, tart cooking apples
- One cup of white all-purpose flour
- Six teaspoons of sugar, divided
- One tsp baking powder
- One huge egg that has been beaten
- one-third cup of One percent skim milk
- one-third cup almond milk
- One teaspoon, or around 3/4 cup, canola oil for deep-fat frying
- half a teaspoon of cinnamon

Instructions

- Core and peel the apples. Each apple should yield five rings that are about 1/2" thick.
- Combine flour, baking powder, and two tablespoons sugar in a mixing dish.
- Mix the egg, milk, almond milk, and one teaspoon of oil in another bowl.
- Blend the dry ingredients with the egg mixture, stirring just until combined.
- Heat 1" of cooking oil to 375° F in a skillet that is at least 2" deep.
- One by one, dip apple slices into batter. Fry until golden brown, about 1 to 1 1/2 minutes, in heated oil. blot with paper towels.
- Sprinkle the remaining 1/4 cup sugar and cinnamon over the fritters. Warm up the food.

Nutritional Facts: Calories 145kcal, Fat 9g, Carbohydrates 15g, Protein 1g, Sodium 33mg, Calcium 30mg Phosphorus 26mg, Potassium 67mg

19. MEXICAN BAKED BEANS & RICE

Cooking time: 1 hr   **Yield:** 4

Ingredients

- Two tsp olive oil
- One little onion, chopped
- One little poblano pepper, chopped
- one sliced garlic clove
- One cup of basmati rice

- two paprika tsp
- One teaspoon of ground cumin
- one teaspoon of dried oregano
- salt and ground black pepper to taste
- two teaspoons tomato paste
- One fourteen-ounce can of washed and drained pinto beans; two cups vegetable broth

Instructions

- In a medium pot set over medium-high heat, warm the olive oil.
- For two to three minutes, cook and sauté the onion, poblano pepper, and garlic in high oil.
- Add the rice and simmer, stirring now and then, for about 2 minutes, or until the rice is fully covered with oil.
- Add oregano, cumin, paprika, salt, and black pepper for seasoning.
- Add the tomato paste and let it cook for a minute or two.
- Add the pinto beans and the vegetable broth. Boil, then turn down the heat. For 15 to 20 minutes, or until the rice is soft, cover and simmer.
- After turning off the heat, cover the pot and leave it to stand for at least five minutes. Using a fork, fluff.

Nutritional Facts: Calories 348kcal, Fat 9g, Carbohydrates 59g, Protein 10g, Sodium 624mg, Calcium 78mg, Potassium 413mg

20. SMOKEY HAM OMELETS

Cooking time: 35 mins   **Yield:** 2

Ingredients

- Four eggs
- chopped half a cup of red pepper
- one-third cup finely chopped onions
- 1/4 cup chopped low-sodium ham (ideally a honey ham)
- One-third tsp smoked paprika
- One or two teaspoons olive oil
- Powdered garlic
- Powdered onion
- Chives choose

Instructions

- In a heated skillet with oil, sauté the onion.
- Add the red pepper once the onions are soft and transparent, and sauté it until the edges start to get a little toasted. Cook the ham and paprika for one to two minutes, or until aromatic.
- To make the omelette, beat the egg with a fork in a bowl. Set your skillet's temperature to medium-low. Add one tablespoon of oil to the heated pan and swirl to coat.
- After adding the egg mixture, wait ten to twenty seconds for it to set. After carefully moving the set eggs to the center of the pan using a heat-safe spatula, tilt the pan to allow the runny eggs to take their position. Continue

doing this until there are almost no runny eggs left to move.

- With a spatula, carefully remove the omelet's bottom from the pan. To make sure the pan is not caught anywhere, tilt it slightly forward and backward.
- Add some onion and garlic powder.
- Spoon one half of the omelet with the smoky ham filling, then fold over.
- Allow it to settle for a short while before moving it from the pan to a platter.
- Add chives as a garnish and savor!

Nutritional Facts: Calories 275kcal, Fat 2g, Carbohydrates 10g, Protein 19g, Sodium 372mg, Calcium 73mg, Potassium 335mg

21. EGG & AVOCADO BAKE

Cooking time: 20 mins   **Yield:** 2

Ingredients

- One avocado, cut in half
- Two big eggs
- freshly ground black pepper to taste
- One tablespoon of finely chopped parsley

Instructions

- Turn the oven on to 425°F.
- Crack one egg gently, being sure to preserve the yolk, into a small bowl.

- Place the avocado halves cut-side up on a baking pan. Divide the egg in half. Continue with the second half of the avocado and egg. Add pepper for seasoning.
- Bake the egg for 15 minutes, or until set. Take out of the oven and top with parsley. Serve.

Nutritional Facts: Calories 239kcal, Fat 20g, Carbohydrates 9g, Protein 9g, Sodium 84mg, Calcium 43mg. Phosphorus 160mg, Potassium 571mg

22. CHEESY SCRAMBLED EGGS WITH FRESH HERBS

Cooking time: 35 mins   **Yield:** 4

Ingredients

- Three eggs, room temperature
- Two yolks, room temperature
- ½ cup room temperature cream cheese
- ¼ cup rice milk without sugar
- One tablespoon of finely chopped green portion alone of a scallion
- One tablespoon of freshly chopped tarragon
- Twice as much unsalted butter
- freshly ground peppercorns, according to taste

Instructions

- The eggs, egg whites, cream cheese, rice milk, scallions, and tarragon should all be thoroughly mixed and smoothed out in a medium-sized bowl.
- Melt the butter in a large skillet over medium-high heat, swirling to coat the pan evenly.
- Add the egg mixture and simmer, stirring, until the curds are creamy and the eggs are thick, about 5 minutes. Add pepper for seasoning.

Nutritional Facts: Calories 221kcal, Fat 19g, Carbohydrates 3g, Protein 8g, Sodium 192mg, Calcium 72mg. Phosphorus 118mg, Potassium 139mg

23. PINEAPPLE BREAD

Cooking time: 40 mins   **Yield:** 15 slices

Ingredients

- one-third cup of unsalted butter
- one cup of pineapple juiced and crushed.
- Six cherries from Maraschino
- Two large eggs
- 1/3 cup of sugar
- 2-1/4 cups flour for all purposes
- One-third tsp baking powder

Instructions

1. Let butter soften outside. Take the pineapple's seeds out. Chop the cherries.

2. Beat butter and sugar together with a mixer until frothy and light. Mix thoroughly after adding the eggs.
3. Combine the flour and baking powder.
4. Blend the flour and sugar ingredients together. Mix in the pineapple and cherries after adding them. Fill a 9 x 5-inch pan that has been buttered. Bake for one hour at 350°F.
5. Remove the loaf from the pan and place it on a wire rack to cool after 10 minutes of cooling. Cut in fifteen slices.

Nutritional Facts: Calories 150kcal, Fat 5g, Carbohydrates 23g, Protein 3g, Sodium 108mg, Calcium 65mg. Phosphorus 56mg, Potassium 52mg

24. BREAKFAST BURRITO WITH GREEN CHILES

Cooking time: 30 mins   **Yield:** 2

Ingredients

- nonstick cooking spray
- Four eggs
- Three teaspoons of chopped Ortega green chilies
- 1/4 tsp ground cumin
- Half a teaspoon of spicy sauce
- two burrito-size flour tortillas

Instructions

- Apply nonstick cooking spray to a medium-sized pan and place it over medium heat.
- Beat eggs, cumin, spicy sauce, and green chilies in a bowl. Once the eggs are cooked, pour them into a skillet and cook, stirring, for one to two minutes.
- In a separate skillet set over medium heat, or for 20 seconds in the microwave, reheat the tortillas. Spoon half of the egg mixture onto each tortilla, then roll each one like a burrito.

Nutritional Facts: Calories 366kcal, Fat 18g, Carbohydrates 33g, Protein 18g, Sodium 594mg, Calcium 117mg. Phosphorus 300mg, Potassium 245mg

25. MUSHROOM AND RED PEPPER OMELET

Cooking time: 25 mins   **Yield:** 1/2

Ingredients

- Half a cup of raw mushroom chunks
- two tablespoons of onion
- 1/4 cup of sweet red peppers in a can
- two tsp of butter
- Three big eggs
- One tsp of Worcestershire sauce
- Two tablespoons of cream cheese whipped
- 1/4 tsp black pepper

Instructions

- Chop the red peppers, onions, and mushrooms.
- One teaspoon of butter should be melted over medium heat in a skillet. Add the onion and mushrooms, and sauté for 5 minutes, or until the onion is soft. Add diced red pepper and stir. After taking the veggies out of the skillet, set them aside.
- In the skillet, melt the last teaspoon of butter. Stir Worcestershire sauce into beaten eggs and simmer over medium heat. Shake the pan to allow the uncooked egg to run underneath the cooked egg, then gently lift the sides of the omelet to cook it evenly.
- Place the veggie mixture on top of the half cooked eggs. Top veggies with dollops of whipped cream cheese. Cook the eggs until they set.
- After taking the skillet off the burner, fold the omelet in half. Add a little pepper. After dividing into two parts, serve.

Nutritional Facts: Calories 199kcal, Fat 15g, Carbohydrates 4g, Protein 11g, Sodium 276mg, Calcium 55mg. Phosphorus 167mg, Potassium 228mg

26. BRAN BREAKFAST BARS

Cooking time: 50 mins   **Yield:** 12

Ingredients

- One cup of water that is boiling
- 1/3 cup of finely chopped raisins or medium-cut dates
- One cup of oatmeal
- Half a cup of whole wheat flour
- 1/3 cup of oil (safflower, soybean, or corn)
- one and a half cups uncooked bran
- Three tsp of brown sugar

Instructions

- Add boiling water to the chopped fruit.
- Give it a minimum of 20 minutes to stand.
- Mix the dry ingredients together in a big bowl.
- After draining the fruit, prepare one cup of the liquid by adding boiling water, then place the liquid in a blender with oil.
- Blend for one minute.
- Pour right away into dry ingredients and stir thoroughly.
- Mix in the fruit.
- Pour batter into an 8 x 10 nonstick baking dish.
- Mark cuttings: 4 rows for the narrow way and 6 rows for the long way after leveling with your fingertips or a spatula.
- Bake for 22 minutes at 375°F in a preheated oven.
- Chill on the rack.
- If storing for more than two days, refrigerate or freeze.

Nutritional Facts: Calories 157kcal, Carbohydrates 23g, Protein 4g, Sodium 3mg, Phosphorus 86mg, Potassium 121mg

27. APPLE SPICE MUFFINS

Cooking time: 40 mins   **Yield:** 12 muffins

Ingredients

- One cup of sugar
- one-third cup canola oil
- Two big eggs
- half a teaspoon of cinnamon powder
- half a teaspoon of ginger powder
- half a teaspoon of powdered cloves
- Half a teaspoon of nutmeg
- One teaspoon baking soda
- 1/4 teaspoon salt
- One cup of plain applesauce
- Two cups of all-purpose flour
- One medium apple

Instructions

- Set oven temperature to 325°F.
- Use nonstick cooking spray to grease a muffin pan.
- Cream together the eggs, oil, and sugar.
- Blend in applesauce, baking soda, salt, and spices.

- Add the flour and stir until a thick batter forms.
- Cut the apple into small pieces using a knife or dicer; peel it if you choose.
- If you're using slices, fill each muffin tin halfway with batter, arrange the pieces, and then top with extra batter. If using bits of apple, mix them into the batter before filling the muffin tray.
- Bake until firm to the touch, 25 to 30 minutes. Take out of the oven and let cool.

Nutritional Facts: Calories 223kcal, Fat 7g, Carbohydrates 37g, Protein 3g, Sodium 159mg, Calcium 12mg. Phosphorus 42mg, Potassium 68mg

28. BUCKWHEAT PANCAKES

Cooking time: 25mins   **Yield:** 4

Ingredients

- 1¾ cups rice milk without sugar
- Two tsp white vinegar
- One cup of buckwheat flour
- ½ cup flour for all purposes
- One spoonful of sugar
- Two tsp baking powder (refer to the tip)
- One big egg
- One tsp vanilla essence
- Divide the two tablespoons of butter for the skillet.

Instructions

- Combine the vinegar and rice milk in a small bowl. Give it a five-minute sit.
- In the meantime, combine the all-purpose flour and buckwheat flour in a big basin. Stir to combine the baking powder and sugar.
- Stir the rice milk with the egg and vanilla until well combined. Mix the dry ingredients with the wet ones until they are well combined.
- Melt 1½ tsp butter in a large skillet over medium heat. Spoon the batter into the skillet using a ¼-cup measuring cup. Cook for 2 to 3 minutes, or until the pancakes start to develop little bubbles on top. After flipping, cook for one to two minutes on the other side.
- After transferring the pancakes to a serving tray, cook the remaining batter in the skillet in batches, using extra butter as necessary.

Nutritional Facts: Calories 281kcal, Fat 9g, Carbohydrates 43g, Protein 7g, Sodium 167mg, Calcium 148mg. Phosphorus 199mg, Potassium 241mg

29. CHEESESTEAK QUICHE

Cooking time: 60 mins   **Yield:** 6

Ingredients

- One cup of diced onions
- one-third of a pound of shaved sirloin steak meat
- two teaspoons of canola oil
- ½ cup shredded pepper jack cheese, five beaten eggs, and one cup cream
- 1" x 9" prepared pie crust, deep par-cooked
- ½ teaspoon of black pepper, ground

Instructions

- Cut the steak into rough pieces after shaving.
- In a sauté pan with oil, cook chopped steak and onions until the meat is well browned. Allow it to cool down for ten minutes. Add cheese, fold, and set aside.
- Beat the cream and eggs with the black pepper in a big basin until well combined.
- Line the bottom of the par-baked pie crust with the steak and cheese mixture. Cover with the egg mixture and bake for 30 minutes at 350° F.
- Once the cheesesteak quiche is covered, shut off the oven. After 10 minutes, let the quiche set before serving.

Nutritional Facts: Calories 527kcal, Fat 19g, Carbohydrates 22g, Protein 22g, Sodium 392mg, Calcium mg. Phosphorus 281mg, Potassium 308mg

30. BUTTERMILK PANCAKES

Cooking time: 45mins   **Yield:** 9

Ingredients

- Two cups of all-purpose flour
- One tsp cream of tartar
- one-half tsp baking soda
- two tsp sugar
- Two cups buttermilk (low-fat)
- Two big eggs
- One tablespoon and half a cup of canola oil (for cooking)

Instructions

- Heat a skillet to a medium temperature.
- Mix the dry ingredients together in a big bowl. To the buttermilk, oil, and egg mixture, add the dry ingredients. Blend the dry ingredients with a spoon or whisk until fully moistened.
- Grease the pan with a tablespoon of canola oil. Spoon the pancake batter onto the skillet using a ⅓-cup measuring cup. The width of each pancake should be around 4 inches. To make flipping the pancakes easier, space them about 2" apart. When the bubbles on top of the pancakes have mostly vanished, turn them over with a spatula. When the middle no longer seems damp, let the opposite side brown.

- Proceed to the serving tray.
- Consider serving with a side of eggs and fresh fruit for a healthier twist.

Nutritional Facts: Calories 217kcal, Fat 9g, Carbohydrates 27g, Protein 6g, Sodium 330mg, Calcium 74mg. Phosphorus 100mg, Potassium 182mg

31. 40-SECOND OMELET

Cooking time: 10 mins   **Yield:** 1

Ingredients

- two eggs
- two tsp water
- One tablespoon of butter without salt
- 1/2 cup of filling (seafood, meat, or vegetables)
- Two teaspoons of grated cheese

Instructions

- Whisk eggs and water together.
- Get your fillings ready.
- Heat the butter in a 10-inch omelet pan or fry pan, then add the egg mixture.
- To allow uncooked sections to reach the hot pan, carefully move cooked portions from the edges toward the middle. Pan tilt and adjust as needed. Continue until the eggs solidify and stop flowing.
- Add cheese and half of the filling to the omelet.

- Fold the omelet in half using the spatula.
- Accompany with a dollop of Quick Pesto, 60-Second Salsa, or sour cream.

Nutritional Facts: Calories 245kcal, Carbohydrates 1g, Protein 13g, Sodium 145mg, Phosphorus 201mg, Potassium 141mg

32. SOUR CREAM APPLE BREAD

Cooking time: 1hr 40mins   **Yield:** 10 loaves

Ingredients

- nonstick cooking spray
- 1-2/3 cups of all-purpose flour
- one and a half teaspoons of baking powder
- One-fourth teaspoon of baking soda
- half a teaspoon of cinnamon powder
- 1/4 tsp salt
- 1/2 cup of sugar, granulated
- 1/4 cup of canola oil
- two white eggs
- one-third cup applesauce
- two thirds cup low-fat sour cream
- One cup of Granny Smith apples
- Half a cup of confectioners' sugar
- six tsp water

Instructions

- Set oven temperature to 350°F.

- Apply cooking spray to an 8-1/2" x 4-3/4" loaf pan.
- After peeling, cut the Granny Smith apple into 1/4" pieces.
- Mix together flour, salt, baking soda, baking powder, and ground cinnamon. Put away for use at a later time.
- Beat oil and granulated sugar together at medium speed.
- Add the applesauce, egg whites, and flour mixture and beat until well blended.
- Add the apples and sour cream and stir until well mixed.
- Evenly distribute mixture into loaf pan. When a toothpick put into the center comes out clean, bake for 50 to 55 minutes.
- Let cool for 20 minutes on a rack. Take out of the pan and allow to cool.
- Combine water and confectioners' sugar. Pour over the loaf. Cut into ten pieces.

Nutritional Facts: Calories 135kcal, Fat 3g, Carbohydrates 24g, Protein 3g, Sodium 139mg, Calcium 42mg. Phosphorus 48mg, Potassium 74mg

33. STRAWBERRY BREAD

Cooking time: 1hr 15mins   **Yield:** 20

Ingredients

- 14 ounces or 2-1/2 cups fresh strawberries frozen strawberries without extra sugar
- Three cups of white all-purpose flour
- Two cups of powdered sugar
- One tsp baking soda
- 1/4 tsp ground cinnamon
- Salt, 3/4 tsp 4 big eggs
- One cup of canola oil

Instructions

- Set the oven's temperature to 350°F.
- Chop the strawberries finely.
- Beat the eggs in a medium-sized mixing bowl. Stir thoroughly after adding the strawberries and canola oil.
- Combine the dry ingredients in a large separate mixing bowl.
- Pour the egg mixture into the well created in the middle of the dry ingredients.
- Don't overmix; instead, use a large spoon to mix until thoroughly combined.
- Transfer the mixture into a pair of ungreased 9" x 5" bread pans. For 50 to 60 minutes, bake.
- After 15 minutes of cooling, carefully take the bread from the loaf pans by using a knife to loosen the sides. Place to cool on a rack.
- To keep the bread fresh, serve it or cover it with foil or plastic wrap. Loaves may be frozen or chilled.

Nutritional Facts: Calories 254kcal, Fat 12g, Carbohydrates 33g, Protein 3g, Sodium 157mg, Calcium 10mg. Phosphorus 39mg, Potassium 64mg

34. ITALIAN APPLE FRITTERS

Cooking time: 30 mins   **Yield:** 16

Ingredients

- One and a half all-purpose flour
- One and a half-cup of milk or water
- 1/4 tsp kosher salt
- three tsp sugar
- Four apples should be cored, skinned, and cut crosswise into ½-inch slices.
- For frying, use sunflower or peanut oil
- Three teaspoons of powdered sugar to dust
- Three tsp of cinnamon to sprinkle on

Instructions

- In a mixing bowl, whisk together the flour, sugar, salt, and water or milk until a homogeneous batter forms.
- In a deep fryer or a medium pot, heat the oil. Once the oil reaches 350 degrees, thoroughly coat three apple slices in the batter. Then, one by one, drop the slices into the oil and fry them for about three minutes on each side, or until they turn golden. Transfer to a baking sheet covered with parchment paper, and fry the remaining apples in small batches.
- Serve the fried apples right away after dusting them with cinnamon and confectioners sugar.

Nutritional Facts: Calories 145kcal, Fat 9g, Carbohydrates 15g, Protein 1g, Sodium 33mg, Calcium 30mg. Phosphorus 26mg, Potassium 67mg

35. GREEN BEANS WITH TURNIPS

Cooking time: 25mins   **Yield:** 1

Ingredients

- One pound of recently harvested green beans
- two medium turnips
- two cloves of garlic
- One tablespoon of butter without salt
- half a teaspoon of pepper, black
- 1/4 tsp salt
- One-fourth teaspoon of paprika

Instructions

- Slice the green beans into 1-1/2-inch slices after removing the ends. After peeling, cut turnips into eight equal pieces. Dice the cloves of garlic.
- Put the garlic and veggies in a medium saucepan. Put three cups of water on top and come to a boil. For fifteen minutes, cook uncovered at medium heat.

- Once the saucepan is off the heat, empty the water. Add salt, pepper, and butter. Toss gently to combine vegetables and seasonings. Warm up the food.
- Transfer to a serving platter and top with paprika.

Nutritional Facts: Calories 58kcal, Fat 3g, Carbohydrates 7g, Protein 1g, Sodium 104mg, Calcium 36mg. Phosphorus 33mg, Potassium 199mg

36. BURRITOS RÁPIDOS

Cooking time: 20 mins   **Yield:** 2

Ingredients

- 1 1/2 tsp olive or canola oil
- ½ red bell pepper, chopped
- 4 thinly sliced green onions (scallions)
- Four 6-inch corn tortillas and eight beaten eggs
- One teaspoon of optional chili powder
- One spoonful of cheese, if desired

Instructions

- In a medium nonstick frying pan, heat the oil over medium heat.
- Add the bell pepper and green onion, and simmer for 3 minutes or until softened.
- Add the eggs and scramble for three to five minutes, or until the eggs are fully

cooked. When finished, they ought to appear somewhat damp.
- After putting the tortillas on a platter, sandwich them between two wet paper towels.
- Tortillas should be microwaved for 2 minutes.
- Fill warm tortillas with egg mixture.
- Enjoy after rolling up the tortillas.

Nutritional Facts: Calories 229kcal, Fat 13g, Carbohydrates 13g, Protein 14g, Sodium 137mg, Calcium 77mg. Phosphorus 254mg, Potassium 211mg

37. EGG FRIED RICE

Cooking time: 10 mins   **Yield:** 10

Ingredients

- Two tsp of black sesame oil
- Two ovum and two whites
- One tablespoon of canola oil
- One cup of sprouting beans
- ⅓ cup finely chopped green onions
- 4 cups cold cooked rice
- 1/4 cup defrosted frozen peas
- ¼ teaspoon freshly ground black pepper

Instructions

- In a small bowl, mix together the eggs, egg whites, and sesame oil. After giving it a good stir, set it aside.

- In a big nonstick skillet, heat canola oil over medium-high heat.
- Stir-fry the egg mixture until it's done.
- Add the green onions and bean sprouts. For two minutes, stir-fry.
- Add the peas and rice. Stir-fry until everything is well heated.
- Add black pepper for seasoning, then serve right away.

Nutritional Facts: Calories 137kcal, Fat 4g, Carbohydrates 21g, Protein 5g, Sodium 38mg, Calcium 20mg. Phosphorus 67mg, Potassium 89mg

38. LAKSA

Cooking time: 20 mins   **Yield:** 4

Ingredients

- Twelve peeled and deveined prawns
- Three tablespoons of reduced-salt Laksa paste
- Noodles Vermicelli, 300g
- One medium-sized pepper
- One medium-sized bok choy
- One cup of green beans
- 400 milliliters of coconut milk

Instructions

- Vermicelli noodles should be soaked in hot water until tender, then drained and set aside.

- Add the coconut milk and one cup of water to the saucepan with the Laksa paste and heat over medium heat until aromatic. Heat till boiling.
- Green beans, capsicum, and bok choy should all be added to the saucepan.
- Stir in noodles and prawns. Simmer for three to five minutes.
- Warm up and serve.

Nutritional Facts: Carbohydrates 27g, Protein 12g, Sodium 611mg, Phosphate 167mg, Potassium 577mg

39. ASPARAGUS BACON HASH

Cooking time: 15 mins   **Yield:** 1

Ingredients

- 2 to 3 pieces of uncured bacon (around 150 calories)
- One clove of garlic
- 8 ounces of asparagus with cut ends
- 1 ounce of freshly grated Parmesan cheese
- Two big eggs
- Sea salt, red pepper flakes, onion powder, black pepper, and chives, to taste

Instructions

- Fry bacon in a large skillet over medium heat for about 8 minutes, or until crispy.

- While the bacon cooks, chop the asparagus into 2-inch pieces, grate the Parmesan cheese, and crush or slice the garlic.
- Once the bacon is cooked through, remove from heat and place onto a cutting board or plate lined with paper towels. Save the rendered bacon fat.
- Once again, bring the heat back to medium and add the garlic. Stirring occasionally, cook for 30 to 60 seconds or until aromatic.
- Place asparagus in a skillet. Add onion powder, sea salt, and pepper for seasoning, then toss to mix. After cooking for one to two minutes, add some Parmesan cheese.
- Make two holes in the hash with a wooden spoon so that the skillet's bottom is visible. If desired, sprinkle some black pepper on top of each egg after it has been cracked.
- For about four to five minutes, or until the whites are set, cover the skillet and cook. The yolks will remain runny, please note. Cook for a further minute or two if you like your yolks to be firmer.
- Dice the cooked bacon, then add it to the hash along with the red pepper flakes.
- Warm up and serve.

Nutritional Facts: Calories kcal, Fat g, Carbohydrates g, Protein g, Sodium mg, Calcium mg. Phosphorus mg, Potassium mg

40. MAPLE PANCAKES

Cooking time: 30 mins   Yield: 5

Ingredients

- One cup of flour for all purposes
- One spoonful of sugar, granulated
- two tsp baking powder
- One eighth teaspoon salt
- two large egg whites
- One cup low-fat milk (1%).
- Two tsp of canola oil
- One tablespoon of extract from maple

Instructions

- Combine the flour, sugar, baking powder, and salt in a medium-sized mixing bowl. In the middle of the dry mixture, create a well. Put aside.
- Whisk together the egg whites, milk, oil, and maple extract in a sizable mixing basin.
- Pour the entire egg mixture into the dry mixture at once. Mix just until wet; lumps should remain in the batter.
- About 1/4 cup of batter should be added to a hot, lightly greased griddle or heavy skillet to produce 4" pancakes.

- Cook the pancakes for about 2 minutes on each side over medium heat, or until brown. When the pancake's edges are beginning to dry up and its surface is bubbling, flip it. Pancakes should only be turned once and should not be pressed with a spatula to maintain them light and fluffy.

Nutritional Facts: Calories 178kcal, Fat 6g, Carbohydrates 25g, Protein 6g, Sodium 297mg, Calcium 174mg. Phosphorus 116mg, Potassium 126mg

Chapter 5

Lunch Recipes

41. Egg White & Pepper Omelets

Cooking time: 10mins   **Yield:** 1

Ingredients

- Cooking spray
- Four egg whites, or ½ cup of egg whites
- One tablespoon chopped red pepper
- one tablespoon chopped green pepper
- one tablespoon chopped green onion, together with a teaspoon of ground black pepper to taste
- One tablespoon of shredded cheddar cheese

Instructions

- Apply cooking spray to a small nonstick skillet and place it over medium heat.
- Beat the egg whites and then transfer them into a hot pan.
- Top egg whites with peppers and green onions. Add some black pepper, ground. Cook with a lid on for around three to four minutes.
- After adding the cheese, replace the lid and heat for an additional 30 seconds, or until the cheese has melted.
- Slice in half, place on a platter, and savor!

Nutritional Facts: Calories 100kcal, Fat 3g, Carbohydrates 3g, Protein 15g, Sodium 251mg, Calcium 67mg. Phosphorus 57mg, Potassium 258mg

42. Fresh Fruit Compote

Cooking time: 15 mins   **Yield:** 8

Ingredients

- Half a cup of fresh or frozen strawberries
- Half a cup of frozen or fresh blackberries
- Half a cup of fresh or frozen blueberries
- 1/2 cup chopped and pared peaches
- 1/4 cup frozen or fresh red raspberries, sweetened but not thawed
- Half a cup of unsweetened orange juice, either fresh or canned
- One apple, sliced into small bits
- One banana, sliced into small bits

Instructions

- Pour the orange juice into a big jar.
- Add each of the specified components.

- Gently toss.
- Thaw frozen fruit at room temperature for four hours before using.

Nutritional Facts: Calories 44kcal, Fat g, Carbohydrates g, Protein 0.5g, Sodium 1mg, Phosphorus 13mg, Potassium 140mg

43. CILANTRO LIME COD

Cooking time: 20 mins   **Yield:** 4

Ingredients

- one-half cup mayonnaise
- half a cup of raw cilantro
- two tablespoons of lime juice
- One-pound filets of cod

Instructions

- Mix lime juice, chopped cilantro, and mayonnaise in a medium-sized bowl. Spoon 1/4 cup into a small basin and reserve to use as a fish sauce.
- Use the remaining mayonnaise mixture to brush the fish.
- Apply cooking spray to a sizable skillet and place it over medium-high heat. Add the cod filets and cook for 8 minutes, rotating once, or until the fish is firm but still moist. Accompany with a lime-coriander sauce.

Nutritional Facts: Calories 292kcal, Fat 23g, Carbohydrates 1g, Protein 20g, Sodium 228mg, Calcium 14mg. Phosphorus 128mg, Potassium 237mg

44. GINGER SPICED LAMB CHOPS

Cooking time: 23 mins + 1hr   **Yield:** 4

Ingredients

- Two tsp olive oil
- One-third cup low-sodium soy sauce
- One tablespoon of freshly grated and peeled ginger
- one teaspoon finely chopped garlic
- ½ teaspoon powdered chipotle chiles
- A little teaspoon of freshly ground black pepper
- Four 3-oz lamb chops
- One tablespoon of freshly cut cilantro

Instructions

- Mix the olive oil, soy sauce, pepper, ginger, garlic, and chipotle chili powder in a medium-sized bowl.
- Turn to coat after adding the lamb chunks.
- After putting the bowl in the fridge, marinate the chops for an hour, flipping them over a few times.
- Set one of the racks in the upper third of the oven and preheat to broil.
- Lay a baking sheet with a wire rack inside, then place the chops on the rack.

57

- For approximately eight minutes in total, broil the chops, turning them once, until they are medium-done and browned.
- Sprinkle some cilantro over top and serve.

Nutritional Facts: Calories 171kcal, Fat 10g, Carbohydrates 1g, Protein 18g, Sodium 210mg, Calcium 18mg. Phosphorus 173mg, Potassium 298mg

45. SHRIMP IN GARLIC SAUCE (HIGH PROTEIN)

Cooking time: 25 mins   **Yield:** 4

Ingredients

- Eight ounces of raw bowtie pasta
- Three tsp unsalted butter
- three cloves of garlic
- 1/4 cup finely chopped onions
- One pound of uncooked shrimp
- Half a cup of whipped cream cheese
- 1/4 cup of creamer, half and half
- one-fourth cup white wine
- two tsp fresh basil
- one-eighth teaspoon of black pepper

Instructions

- Devein and shell shrimp.
- In a big pot, bring three quarts of water to a boil. After cooking for 12 minutes

with 3 cups of dried bowtie pasta, drain.
- Mince onion and garlic while pasta is boiling. In a skillet over medium heat, melt the butter. Sauté the onion and garlic for one minute. Add shrimp and simmer for 1 to 2 minutes, or until it turns orange; take care not to overcook.
- Take out of the skillet and place the shrimp aside. Turn down the heat. To prepare a sauce, add cream cheese to the skillet and whisk in the butter, onion, and garlic.
- Stir in the half-and-half creamer. Blend the wine in until it's smooth. After cooking, add the shrimp back to the sauce and swirl to coat.
- Place the drained pasta onto four dishes, then add the shrimp and garlic sauce on top. Add a half-tsp of finely chopped fresh basil and black pepper for seasoning.

Nutritional Facts: Calories 483kcal, Fat 14g, Carbohydrates 46g, Protein 32g, Sodium 213mg, Calcium 133mg. Phosphorus 398mg, Potassium 514mg

46. RATATOUILLE

Cooking time: 35mins   **Yield:** 16

Ingredients

- two cups of onions
- Two cups of squashed zucchini
- Three cups of crookneck yellow squash
- One medium eggplant
- two medium-sized carrots
- One bell pepper, green
- One bell pepper, yellow
- one bell pepper, red
- Four cloves of garlic
- Two tsp olive oil
- one cup of tomatoes in cans
- One tablespoon of new basil
- One-third cup of raw oregano
- One tablespoon of newly chopped rosemary
- One teaspoon of new thyme
- One tablespoon of recently harvested sage
- One tablespoon of pepper, black
- Grated Parmesan cheese, eight tablespoons

Instructions

- Chop the peppers, onions, squash, and eggplant. Dice the cloves of garlic. Add carrots, garlic, herbs, black pepper, and canola or olive oil to a big skillet.
- After two minutes of cooking, add the remaining vegetables—aside from the tomatoes.

- Cook the vegetables for ten to fifteen minutes, stirring often, or until they are almost soft.
- Stir in tomatoes and Parmesan cheese.
- Simmer, covered, for about 30 minutes.

Nutritional Facts: Calories 54kcal, Fat 3g, Carbohydrates 6g, Protein 3g, Sodium 84mg, Calcium 57mg. Phosphorus 58mg, Potassium 302mg

47. BEEF & SWEET POTATO BURGERS

Cooking time: mins   **Yield:** 6

Ingredients

- 250g of beef mince
- 350g of sweet potato
- 15g of flat leaf parsley diced finely
- 1 medium zucchini grated
- 2 garlic cloves minced
- 1 egg, gently beated
- Six rolls of hamburgers
- Three cups of finely chopped lettuce
- To serve, cut one onion, half a cucumber, slice one capsicum, and chop some mayonnaise.

Instructions

- Mix thoroughly the beef, sweet potato, parsley, zucchini, garlic, and egg.

- Using a little plain flour on your hands to help, form 6 patties.
- Cook in a frying pan with a drizzle of olive oil over medium heat for 5 minutes on each side.
- Place patties and additional ingredients into each hamburger bun to make burgers.

Nutritional Facts: Carbohydrates 48g, Sodium 414mg, Phosphorus 248mg, Potassium 644mg

48. SHRIMP QUESADILLA

Cooking time: 30 mins   **Yield:** 2

Ingredients

- Five ounces of raw shrimp
- two tsp of cilantro
- One tablespoon of lemon juice
- 1/4 tsp ground cumin
- one-eighth teaspoon of cayenne
- two burrito-size flour tortillas
- Two tsp of sour cream
- four tsp of salsa
- Two tablespoons of cheddar cheese with jalapeño shreds

Instructions

- Devein and shell shrimp. After rinsing, chop into small pieces. Finely chop the cilantro.
- To make the marinade, place the cilantro, lemon juice, cumin, and cayenne pepper in a zip-lock bag. Add the shrimp pieces, then marinade them for five minutes.
- Place the shrimp with marinade in a pan over medium heat. Fry the shrimp for one to two minutes, or until it becomes orange. Turn off the heat and carefully scoop out the shrimp, discarding the marinade.
- Stir the sour cream into the skillet marinade until well combined.
- Use a big skillet or the microwave to reheat tortillas. Top each tortilla with two tsp of salsa. Add half of the shrimp mixture on top, then top with one tablespoon of cheese.
- Top shrimp with 1 tablespoon of the sour cream marinade mixture. After folding the tortilla in half, heat it up in the skillet and take it out. Continue with the second tortilla, the remaining cheese, marinade, and shrimp.
- Divide each tortilla into four parts. When ready to serve, garnish with a wedge of lemon and some cilantro.

Nutritional Facts: Calories 318kcal, Fat 15g, Carbohydrates 26g, Protein 20g, Sodium 398mg, Calcium 139mg. Phosphorus 243mg, Potassium 276mg

49. SAUTEED GREEN BEANS

Cooking time: 20 mins   **Yield:** 4

Ingredients

- 1 ½ cups of frozen green beans, thawed (the salt level of canned beans may increase).
- fat-free cooking spray
- One small yellow onion, chopped
- one garlic clove, minced
- four tablespoons of fake bacon bits
- One-half teaspoon of cayenne

Instructions

- Green beans should be steamed for three minutes or until soft.
- Steam the beans while you sauté the onions and garlic in a big skillet sprayed with cooking spray.
- Add the cayenne pepper, bacon bits, and green beans and stir. Warm up thoroughly.
- Warm up and serve.

Nutritional Facts: Calories 50kcal, Fat 1g, Carbohydrates 7g, Protein 3g, Sodium 136mg, Calcium 41mg. Phosphorus 53mg, Potassium 226mg

50. SLOW COOKER ROAST BEEF

Cooking time: 8 hrs   **Yield:** 10

Ingredients

- One tablespoon of olive oil
- 2.5 pound boneless bottom blade roast
- two cups of chopped carrots
- two cups finely chopped yellow onions
- One cup of cut celery stalks
- four chopped garlic cloves
- One teaspoon pepper

Broth

- ¼ cup balsamic vinegar
- ¼ cup unsalted beef broth
- Two tablespoons of honey

Thickener (Optional)

- Three tablespoons of cornstarch
- Three tablespoons of water

Instructions

- While preparing the veggies, take the piece of meat out of the refrigerator, unpack it, and let it sit at room temperature.
- Place a skillet over medium-high heat and add the olive oil. Sear the meat for a few minutes on each side once the oil is hot.
- Put all the vegetables in the slow cooker's bottom and stir to coat them. After that, arrange the meat piece on top of the veggies in the slow cooker.
- Blend the honey, balsamic vinegar, and beef broth together in a bowl. Next, cover the meat with the broth.

- Combine the liquid honey, balsamic vinegar, and unsalted beef broth in a bowl. Next, cover the meat with the broth.
- Dust the meat with ground black pepper and sliced garlic.
- Set your slow cooker to cook for seven hours at a low temperature.

Optional

- You can utilize the meat just as it is after it is done cooking. The following stages, which are optional, show you how to cut the meat so that it can be served with its thickened broth.
- The piece of beef must first be taken out of the slow cooker and placed aside for the time being in order to accomplish this.
- Combine the cornstarch and water in a glass. Finally, stir in the slow cooker's broth.
- Put the meat back in the slow cooker and set the timer for 30 minutes at high heat. Simmer somewhat covered, then serve when cooled slightly.

Nutritional Facts: Calories 250kcal, Fat 13g, Carbohydrates 14g, Protein 20g, Sodium 116mg, Calcium 45mg. Phosphorus 215mg, Potassium 514mg

51.ZUCCHINI BREAD

Cooking time: 1hr 15mins   **Yield:** 16

slices

Ingredients

- three eggs
- 1/4 cup sugar
- One cup of applesauce
- Two cups of shredded, unpeeled zucchini
- One tsp vanilla essence
- ¼ teaspoon baking powder
- 2 cups of flour
- One tsp baking soda
- One tsp of cinnamon
- One-half teaspoon of ginger
- one cup chopped unsalted almonds

Instructions

- Beat the eggs.
- Beat eggs with sugar, applesauce, zucchini, and vanilla.
- Add the dry ingredients to the mixture after sifting them.
- Transfer into a loaf pan and bake for one hour at 375°F.
- Cut into sixteen pieces.

Nutritional Facts: Calories 200kcal, Fat g, Carbohydrates 33.2g, Protein 4.4g, Sodium 100mg, Calcium 24mg. Phosphorus 78mg, Potassium 128mg

52.ZUCCHINI FRITTATA

Cooking time: 25 mins   **Yield:** 9

Ingredients

- two medium-sized zucchini
- One medium onion
- 1/4 cup parsley and 1 clove of garlic
- Four big eggs
- one cup of baking mix for biscuits
- Grated Parmesan cheese, half a cup
- 1/4 cup of canola oil
- Half a teaspoon of dried marjoram
- 1/4 tsp black pepper

Instructions

- Set oven temperature to 350°F. Mince the garlic; chop the parsley and onion; and grate the zucchini. Gently whisk the eggs.
- Mix all the ingredients thoroughly in a sizable basin.
- Pour into a 9-inch cast iron skillet or an 11-by-7-inch pan that has been oiled. Bake until firm and light golden, about 30 to 35 minutes.
- Once cut into nine pieces, serve.

Nutritional Facts: Calories 180kcal, Fat 12g, Carbohydrates 12g, Protein 6g, Sodium 287mg, Calcium 88mg. Phosphorus 172mg, Potassium 203mg

53. LEMON AND BERRY BREAD

Cooking time: 1hr

Ingredients

- 1-1/2 cups white flour, for all purposes
- One tsp baking powder
- one-third cup canola oil
- 2/3 cup of white sugar, granulated
- Two tsp lemon essence
- Four beaten egg whites
- half a cup One percent skim milk
- One cup of raw blueberries
- 3/4 cup of sugar, powdered
- one-fourth cup lemon juice
- One tablespoon of finely chopped lemon peel

Instructions

- Set oven temperature to 350°F. Grease a 9 x 5-inch loaf pan and then sprinkle with flour.
- Mix the flour and baking powder together in a big bowl.
- Combine the egg whites, milk, granulated sugar, lemon extract, and oil in a separate basin.
- Combine flour mixture with sugar and oil mixture. Mix just enough to combine; do not overmix.
- Stir in lemon peel and blueberries.
- Loaf pan should be filled with batter, then baked for 40 to 50 minutes, or until the toothpick inserted into the center comes out clean.
- While the bread is baking, make the glaze. Lemon juice and powdered sugar should be combined in a small pot. After the sugar dissolves, heat.

- As soon as the bread comes out of the oven, pierce it with a 1-inch hole every time, then cover it with a lemon glaze.

Nutritional Facts: Calories 212kcal, Fat 7g, Carbohydrates 34g, Protein 3g, Sodium 54mg, Calcium 46mg. Phosphorus 68mg, Potassium 66mg

54. GOLDEN POTATO CROQUETTES

Cooking time: 40mins   **Yield:** 2

Ingredients

- Low-potassium potatoes prepared according to a low-potassium recipe - One pound, or 400 grams 25g (1 oz) of mashed unsalted butter
- milk - one-half cup
- salt - one-fourth teaspoon
- black pepper - one-fourth teaspoon
- egg - one-half medium-sized, freshly beaten
- white breadcrumbs - 90g (3½ oz)
- olive oil (about 3 tablespoons) for frying

Instructions

- Follow the Low Potassium Vegetables recipe to cook the potatoes.
- In a bowl, combine the cooked low-potassium potatoes, butter, milk, and spices. Mash.

- Using your hands, form the croquette and then dip it into the beaten egg.
- Coat every croquette with the crumbs.
- When a little olive oil is heated, add the croquettes to the pan one at a time, being careful to provide enough space for you to be able to turn them easily.
- Fry until golden and crisp on all sides. Hold warm until everyone is ready.

Nutritional Facts: Calories 570kcal, Fat 30g, Carbohydrates 70g, Protein 10g, Sodium 1.2g, Phosphate 157mg, Potassium 398mg

55. THAI CHICKEN CURRY

Cooking time: 30 mins   **Yield:** 4

Ingredients

- One tablespoon of canola oil
- Cut one pound of chicken breast into cubes
- ½ cup finely chopped onion
- 2 teaspoons red curry paste
- three sliced garlic cloves,
- one tablespoon minced fresh ginger,
- One chopped lime juice
- half a cup of chopped red pepper
- One cup chicken broth, unsalted
- ten freshly sliced basil leaves
- One tablespoon of cornflour
- One tablespoon of water
- one-third cup of plain yogurt

Instructions

- Heat the oil in a nonstick frying pan over medium heat. Add the onion and fry the chicken until it begins to lightly brown.
- Stir together the diced peppers, diced garlic, ginger, lime juice, and curry paste.
- Add the basil and the chicken broth. Simmer for five minutes.
- Stir the cornstarch into the pan after diluting it with one tablespoon of water. Simmer the sauce until it thickens.
- After turning off the heat, add the yogurt to the pan.
- Enjoy with basmati rice after serving!

Nutritional Facts: Calories 224kcal, Fat 8g, Carbohydrates 10g, Protein 28g, Sodium 82mg, Calcium 59mg. Phosphorus 304mg, Potassium 588mg

56. ROASTED TURKEY BREAST WITH SALT-FREE HERB SEASONING

Cooking time: 45 mins   **Yield:** 10

Ingredients

- 3 pounds of fresh, skin-on, bone-in turkey breast halves
- 1/4 cup of butter
- One tablespoon of a herb seasoning combination without salt
- one-fourth cup onion

Instructions

- Set the oven's temperature to 350ºC.
- Chop the onion finely. Add the onion and herb seasoning blend to the melted butter. Split the mixture in half.
- With the skin side down, lay the turkey breast in a large roasting pan or skillet. Apply a single tablespoon of the spice blend on top.
- Using your fingers, turn the breast over and loo0sen the skin. Spoon 3 tablespoons of the spice mixture over the skin and meat. Attach the skin's borders to the breast meat with toothpicks.
- Bake the pan for an hour in the oven.
- After taking the pan out of the oven, cover the turkey skin with the leftover spice mixture.
- After 15 to 20 minutes, or when the meat thermometer registers 160 degrees Fahrenheit, return the pan to the oven.
- Before slicing, take the pan out of the oven and give the turkey breast ten to fifteen minutes to rest.

Nutritional Facts: Calories 203kcal, Fat 11g, Carbohydrates 1g, Protein 25g, Sodium 88mg, Calcium 20mg, Phosphorus 184mg, Potassium 265mg

57. CLASSIC BEEF STROGANOFF WITH EGG NOODLES

Cooking time: 50 mins   **Yield:** 6

Ingredients

- One cup of finely chopped onions
- One beaten egg
- Two tablespoons of low-sodium French's® Worcestershire sauce
- 1/4 cup of breadcrumbs
- One spoonful of mayonnaise
- One spoonful of tomato sauce without additional salt
- One pound of ground beef
- Three tsp canola oil
- two tsp of flour
- three cups of water
- one tsp finely ground black pepper
- Four tsp Superior to Bouillon® beef with lower salt content
- half a cup of sour cream
- Two tablespoons of chives
- One-half package (12 ounces) of cooked broad egg noodles
- Two tablespoons of chilled, diced, unsalted butter
- 1/4 cup parsley
- One tablespoon of finely chopped rosemary

Instructions

- Combine the first six ingredients and half of the black pepper in a large bowl. Stir in the ground meat. Form 16 meatballs of the same size.
- Meatballs from stroganoff should be cooked in a big sauté pan over medium heat until browned. After moving all of the meatballs to one side, thoroughly combine the flour and oil in the pan. After adding the water, bouillon, and the remaining black pepper, stir until the mixture thickens, about ten minutes.
- After removing from the heat and mixing in the sour cream and chives, serve with egg noodles.
- Pasta
- When the egg noodles are warm, add them to a saucepan or big sauté pan with two tablespoons of water, mix, and turn off the heat. Add butter, parsley, and rosemary, and stir until well combined.

Nutritional Facts: Calories 490kcal, Fat 32g, Carbohydrates 30g, Protein 20g, Sodium 598mg, Calcium 56mg. Phosphorus 230mg, Potassium 423mg

58. DIJON SALMON WITH GREEN BEAN PILAF

Cooking time: 30 mins   **Yield:** 4

Ingredients

- 1¼ pounds of peeled and divided into four parts of wild salmon
- Three tablespoons, divided, of extra virgin olive oil
- one tablespoon of finely chopped garlic
- One-fourth teaspoon of salt
- Mayonnaise, two tablespoons
- Half a tsp whole-grain mustard
- Half a teaspoon of ground pepper, split
- Twelve ounces of thin green beans, or haricots verts, pre trimmed and divided into thirds
- One little lemon, squeezed and divided into four wedges
- Two tsp of pine nuts
- One 8-oz container of already cooked brown rice
- two tsp water
- freshly chopped parsley as a garnish

Instructions

- Turn the oven on to 425°F. Put parchment paper or foil around the edge of a baking pan.
- Place fish on the baking sheet that has been preheated and brush with 1 tablespoon oil. Using the side of a chef's knife or a fork, mash the garlic and salt into a paste. In a separate bowl, mix 1/4 teaspoon pepper, mustard, and mayonnaise with a scant teaspoon of the garlic paste. Cover the fish with the mixture.
- Roast the salmon for 6 to 8 minutes per inch of thickness, or until the thickest section flakes readily with a fork.
- In the meantime, bring a large skillet filled with the remaining 2 tablespoons of oil to a medium-high heat. Stir in the green beans, pine nuts, lemon zest, remaining garlic paste, and 1/4 teaspoon pepper. Cook, stirring, for 2 to 4 minutes, or until the beans are just soft. Turn down the heat to medium. When the rice is heated, add the water and stir-fry it for an additional two to three minutes.
- If preferred, garnish the salmon with parsley and serve it with lemon wedges and green bean pilaf.

Nutritional Facts: Calories 442kcal, Fat 24.8g, Carbohydrates 21.6g, Protein 32.2g, Sodium 605mg, Calcium 99mg. Phosphorus 500mg, Potassium 706mg

59. SHISH KEBABS

Cooking time: 30 mins   **Yield: 6**

Ingredients

- Half a cup of pure white vinegar
- half a cup of canola oil
- 1/4 tsp black pepper
- one-fourth teaspoon powdered garlic

- Half a teaspoon of oregano
- 1.5 pounds of sirloin beef
- two medium-sized onions
- Two bell peppers, green
- One red bell pepper

Instructions

- To prepare a marinade, mix together the vinegar, oil, pepper, garlic powder, and oregano.
- Cube the beef, measuring 1-1/2". Chop the bell peppers into 1-1/2" squares and the onions into quarters.
- For at least half an hour, marinate the meat and veggies in a closed container.
- Alternate between adding meat and veggies on the skewers.
- Kebabs should be cooked over a medium heat source for 10 to 30 minutes, or until done to your preference.

Nutritional Facts: Calories 358kcal, Fat 26g, Carbohydrates 5g, Protein 26g, Sodium 60mg, Calcium 25mg. Phosphorus 217mg, Potassium 458mg

60. GOBI CURRY

Cooking time: 20 mins   **Yield:** 4

Ingredients

- Twice as much unsalted butter
- 1/2 medium yellow onion, cut finely

- one tsp finely chopped fresh ginger
- half a teaspoon of turmeric
- 1/8 teaspoon of optional cayenne
- One tsp garam masala
- two cups florets of cauliflower
- half a cup of frozen peas
- One tablespoon of water

Instructions

- Melt butter in a medium skillet over medium heat, then add onions and simmer until soft and gently browned—a process known as caramelization.
- Add the garam masala, ginger, turmeric, and cayenne pepper and stir.
- Add peas and cauliflower and stir.
- Cover after adding water.
- After lowering the heat to low, steam for ten minutes.

Nutritional Facts: Calories 58kcal, Carbohydrates 5g, Protein 2g, Sodium 25mg, Phosphorus 27mg, Potassium 152mg

61. CREAMY SHRIMP AND BROCCOLI FETTUCCINE

Cooking time: 30 mins   **Yield:** 4

Ingredients

- Four ounces of raw fettuccine
- 1-3/4 cup of florets of broccoli

- Three-quarters of a pound of medium-sized frozen shrimp
- One clove of garlic
- Ten ounces of cream cheese
- half a teaspoon of powdered garlic
- one-fourth cup lemon juice
- one-third teaspoon of ground peppercorns
- 1/4 cup of creamer, half and half
- one-fourth cup red bell pepper

Instructions

- Pasta should be cooked as directed, but without salt.
- For the final three minutes of cooking, add the broccoli. Empty. Stay warm.
- In a large nonstick skillet, sauté and stir shrimp and garlic over medium heat for 2 to 3 minutes, or until shrimp are heated through.
- Stir in half-and-half, cream cheese, lemon juice, crushed peppercorns, and garlic powder. Stir-fry for two minutes.
- Stir in the shrimp mixture and pasta. Add some bell pepper to it.

Nutritional Facts: Calories 468kcal, Fat 28g, Carbohydrates 28g, Protein 27g, Sodium 374mg, Calcium 157mg, Phosphorus 335mg, Potassium 469mg

62. BAKED SEA BASS AND ROASTED RED PEPPER

Cooking time: **Yield**: 4

Ingredients

- Two orange and two red peppers, seeded and chopped into bits
- Eight garlic cloves, cut into three pieces
- Two thinly sliced red chilies
- Four tiny oregano sprigs (or one dried tsp)
- 4 Tbsp, 70 ml olive oil
- 4 × 190g cleaned and descaled sea bass
- 50g of rocket with a black pepper pinch

Instructions

- Set oven temperature to 200°C/gas 6. With one tablespoon of olive oil reserved, arrange the red and yellow peppers and sprinkle with the garlic, chilies, oregano sprigs, and olive oil.
- To ensure consistent cooking, turn the dish halfway through the 40-minute bake. In the meantime, make five to six incisions on each side of the fish, spread the leftover olive oil on the skin, and season with salt and black pepper.
- Set the fish down. Place the dish back in the oven and bake it for an additional 15 minutes, or until the fish is cooked through, rotating the dish

halfway through. Accompany the dish with the rocket and roasted veggies.

Nutritional Facts: Calories 349kcal, Fat 19g, Carbohydrates 11g, Protein 37g, odium 165mg, Calcium 96mg. Phosphorus 471mg, Potassium 623mg

63. OVEN-BAKED CHICKEN THIGHS

Cooking time: 40 mins   **Yield:**2

Ingredients

- Ten ounces of skin-on, bone-in chicken thighs (two thighs)
- one-third cup white wine
- One lemon
- One-third cup of raw oregano
- 1/4 tsp freshly cracked black pepper
- One tablespoon of olive oil

Instructions

- Turn the oven up to 350 degrees.
- Place the chicken thighs in an ovenproof pan with the white wine. Drizzle chicken with half of the lemon. Cut the last lemon into slices, then place them over the chicken.
- Olive oil, cracked pepper, and fresh oregano are used to season chicken.
- Bake the chicken for 25–30 minutes, or until it reaches a temperature of 165–175 degrees Fahrenheit within.

Nutritional Facts: Calories 334kcal, Fat 26g, Carbohydrates 5g, Protein 20g, Sodium 100mg, Calcium 34mg. Phosphorus 198mg, Potassium 328mg

64. SUMMER HARVEST EGG MUFFIN CUPS

Cooking time: 40 mins   **Yield:** 12 muffins

Ingredients

- 1 cup of small-diced or shredded vegetables (we used 1/3 cup each of carrot, yellow squash, and red pepper).
- One tsp oil
- Eight eggs
- One tablespoon of newly chopped herbs We used parsley, basil, and dill.
- Three thinly sliced green onion stalks, both green and white
- two tsp mayonnaise
- Brie not required; thin slices
- 1 tsp. of taste-tested lemon zest

Instructions

- Vegetables should be sautéed in oil until just soft. Put aside to cool. In a bowl, whisk together mayo and eggs. Add the chopped green onions and herbs. Include the cooked vegetables. Spoon mixture into 12 separate muffin pans. Add a tiny piece of brie on top (opt) The finest muffin tins are silicon ones, as they make it easy for the muffins to come out. As an alternative, you might prepare this like a breakfast casserole in a 9x9 dish.

- Bake for 20 to 25 minutes at 350 degrees, or until the middle of each muffin is set. Sprinkle some lemon zest over the top of every muffin.

Nutritional Facts: Calories 66kcal, Fat 4g, Carbohydrates 3g, Protein 5g, Sodium 59mg, Calcium 25mg, Potassium 88mg

65. CHORIZO AND EGG TORTILLA

Cooking time: 25 mins   **Yield:** 1

Ingredients

- 1/4 cup chorizo with low sodium
- One big egg
- Two 6-inch corn tortillas and one

Instructions

- Prepare a quarter-cup quantity. Simple Cook the chorizo in a skillet over medium heat, using a spatula to finely crumble the meat.
- If necessary, drain extra water and fat. Add one egg and whisk to incorporate as the egg cooks, once the meat is cooked through.
- Accompany with two corn tortillas.

Nutritional Facts: Calories 346kcal, Fat 18g, Carbohydrates 25g, Protein 21g,

Sodium 316mg, Calcium 94mg. Phosphorus 278mg, Potassium 397mg

66. VEGAN BOLOGNESE SAUCE

Cooking time: 1hr 5mins   **Yield:** 8

Ingredients

- Dried porcini mushrooms, ½ ounce
- One tablespoon of pure olive oil
- Three tablespoons of plant-based butter
- One onion, chopped finely
- two carrots, cut finely
- two celery stalks, cut finely
- One pound of finely chopped shiitake mushrooms
- One cup of non-dairy milk, such as unsweetened oat milk
- 1/2 tsp finely grated nutmeg
- one cup of white wine, dry
- One 28-oz can of chopped Italian plum tomatoes with their juices
- ¾ cup cooked French lentils, either green or black, following the instructions on the package
- freshly ground peppercorns, according to taste
- Optional: vegan parmesan cheese

Special Equipments

- Dutch oven
- mesh strainer

Instructions

- To prepare the porcini mushrooms, put them in a bowl and soak them for half an hour in warm water.
- Gently remove the mushrooms from the water, being careful not to shake up any dirt or debris that could have dropped to the bowl's bottom, and then coarsely chop. After straining the mushroom water through a fine mesh screen, keep it aside (a coffee filter can also be used for this purpose).
- In a large saucepan, add the onions, butter, and olive oil. Reduce the heat to medium. Add the onion and sauté for about 5 minutes, or until transparent.
- Add the carrot and celery and simmer for about 3 minutes, stirring regularly.
- Add the shiitake and porcini mushrooms, and simmer, stirring periodically, for about 6 minutes or until the mushrooms release their juices and become soft.
- Turn up the heat to medium-high, then add the oat milk, nutmeg, and the conserved mushroom water. Bring to a boil.
- Lower the temperature to medium and simmer, stirring periodically, for approximately 12 minutes, or until the majority of the liquid evaporates.
- When the wine has evaporated, add it and simmer.
- After turning the heat up to medium-high, add the tomatoes along with their juices, and boil.
- The sauce should barely be bubbling after lowering the heat to a gentle simmer. Simmer for about two and a half to three hours, stirring periodically, or until the flavors meld. To avoid burning, add a little water while simmering if necessary.
- Simmer for ten minutes after adding the cooked lentils and pepper to taste.
- If preferred, top with vegan parmesan cheese.
- Accompany with tagliatelle or rigatoni pasta. Limit the amount to one cup, which should include the pasta and sauce.

Nutritional Facts: Calories 45kcal, Fat 2g, Carbohydrates 6g, Protein 2g, Sodium 49mg, Calcium 22mg. Phosphorus 44mg, Potassium 165mg

67. ASIAN BEEF WRAPS

Cooking time: 40 mins   **Yield:** 4

Ingredients

- four cloves of garlic
- One medium-sized cucumber
- One medium-sized red bell pepper
- One pound of ground beef

- One tablespoon of cooking sherry wine
- One spoonful of soy sauce with lower sodium
- Two tsp red chili sauce
- Two tsp of well-packed brown sugar
- one tsp finely chopped ginger
- One tsp dark sesame oil
- 8 pieces of cooked rice in 1 cup entire iceberg lettuce leaves

Instructions

- Dice the garlic. Dice the bell pepper and cucumber.
- In a medium bowl, thoroughly mix the ground meat with the ginger, garlic, sherry, soy sauce, red chili sauce, brown sugar, and brown sugar.
- Put a big nonstick skillet over medium heat after spraying it with nonstick spray.
- Add the meat mixture and heat for about three minutes, breaking it up with a wooden spoon, until it's cooked through.
- Add the sesame oil and stir; reheat.
- Bring the rice to a boil.
- In a bowl, mix the red bell pepper and cucumber.
- Place two teaspoons of rice, 1/4 cup ground beef, and 1/4 cup cucumber/red pepper combination into each lettuce leaf. Enjoy after wrapping!

Nutritional Facts: Calories 308kcal, Fat 15g, Carbohydrates 17g, Protein 26g, Sodium 311mg, Calcium 46mg. Phosphorus 252mg, Potassium 591mg

68. STIR-FRIED GARLIC GREEN BEANS WITH TOASTED ALMONDS

Cooking time: 30 mins   **Yield:** 8

Ingredients

- Three tsp canola oil
- One pound of green beans
- 1/4 cup of almonds, slivered
- two tsp powdered garlic

Instructions

- Turn the heat up to medium-high.
- Toss to evenly coat with oil after adding the green beans.
- Sauté for five minutes.
- Add the garlic powder and almonds.
- Sauté for five minutes.

Nutritional Facts: Calories 91kcal, Carbohydrates 5g, Protein 2g, Sodium 1mg, Phosphorus 25mg, Potassium 171mg

69. TORTILLA BEEF ROLL UPS (HIGH PROTEIN)

Cooking time: 15 mins   Yield: 2

Ingredients

- two 6-inch flour tortillas
- Two tablespoons of cream cheese whipped
- Five ounces of cooked roast beef
- 1/4 cup chopped red onion
- 1/4 sliced red, yellow, or green sweet bell pepper
- Eight slices of cucumber
- Two leaves of romaine lettuce
- One tsp Mrs. Dash® herb spice blend

Instructions

- Spread tortillas with cream cheese.
- Ingredients should be divided in half to produce two tortillas. Arrange the roast beef, red onion, pepper strips, cucumbers, and lettuce in layers on each tortilla.
- Add a dash of Mrs. Dash® Herb Seasoning.
- Like a jelly roll, roll up.
- Serve each tortilla whole, or cut each into four pieces.

Nutritional Facts: Calories 258kcal, Fat 10g, Carbohydrates 18g, Protein 24g, Sodium 279mg, Calcium 59mg. Phosphorus 253mg, Potassium 448mg

70. FISH WITH MUSHROOMS

Cooking time: 30 mins   **Yield:** 4

Ingredients

- One-pound fresh filets of cod
- Two tsp margarine
- 1-1/2 cups of freshly sliced mushrooms
- one-fourth cup white onion
- A single tsp of dried thyme

Instructions

- **Put filets into** a rectangular baking dish that holds two quarts. (Thaw the fish first if using frozen rather than fresh.)
- Set oven temperature to 450°F.
- Finely chop the onion.
- In a small saucepan, melt the margarine. Add the onion and mushrooms, and sauté over medium heat until soft.
- Place a combination of mushrooms over fish.
- Dried thyme should be crushed and sprinkled over fish.
- Fish should be baked, uncovered, for 12 to 15 minutes, or until it flakes.

Nutritional Facts: Calories 155kcal, Fat 7g, Carbohydrates 2g, Protein 21g, Sodium 110mg, Calcium 30mg. Phosphorus 225mg, Potassium 561mg

Chapter 6

Dinner Options

71. Minestrone Soup

Cooking time: 45 mins   **Yield:** 1

Ingredients

- 14-oz Diced Tomatoes with No Added Salt
- a half-cup of dry, elbow-shaped macaroni
- Four cups of low-fat, low-sodium chicken broth
- 1 teaspoon crushed black pepper
- 1 teaspoon dried basil leaves
- One teaspoon of dried oregano leaves
- ½ cup of chopped zucchini
- One huge carrot
- two substantial celery stalks
- two garlic cloves
- ½ big onion
- Two tablespoons of olive oil
- One can of green snap peas without additional salt

Instructions

- Chop the garlic, onion, and zucchini. Cut the carrot into shreds. Use one and a half cups of fresh beans, cut into ½-inch pieces, or rinse the canned green beans.
- In a big pot or Dutch oven, warm up the olive oil over medium heat. When onions are transparent, sauté for two to three minutes.
- Add the zucchini, carrot, celery, and garlic. (If using fresh beans, add green beans). Cook until the vegetables are tender, about 5 minutes.
- Add the black pepper, oregano, basil, and canned green beans.
- Add chicken broth and one can of diced, salt-free tomatoes.
- After bringing to a boil, lower heat to simmer. Simmer for ten minutes.
- Cook the pasta for 8 to 10 minutes, or as directed on the package, after adding it.
- Add a fresh basil sprig as a garnish. Pour into a bowl, then savor!

Nutritional Facts: Calories 144kcal, Fat 4.3g, Carbohydrates 21.9g, Protein 5.9g, Sodium 55.1mg, Calcium 51.3mg. Phosphorus 97.8mg, Potassium 355.2mg

72. Crispy baked cauliflower wings

Cooking time: 60 mins   **Yield:** 5

Ingredients

- Cauliflower Wings

- 1/2 cup all-purpose flour
- 1/2 cup water, and additional as necessary
- two tsp powdered garlic
- One tsp of smoky paprika
- A ¼ teaspoon of pepper and salt each
- One-fourth cup of breadcrumbs
- Cut one medium head of cauliflower into florets.
- Three tablespoons of avocado oil
- Buffalo Sauce
- ¼ cup reduced-sodium hot sauce
- 2 tablespoons melted coconut oil
- A teaspoon or two of maple syrup, to taste
- a tsp of garlic powder

Instructions

- Turn the oven on to 450°F. Use parchment paper to line a baking sheet.
- Combine the flour, water, paprika, garlic powder, salt, and pepper in a large zip-lock bag to create a thin batter. If the batter is too thick, add extra water. It should have the consistency of thin pancake batter.
- Transfer half of the breadcrumbs onto a baking sheet or dish.
- After chopping the cauliflower, place the florets inside the zip-lock bag. To coat the cauliflower in batter, gently shake the sealed zipper bag.
- Cauliflower should be fished out using a spider sieve or tongs, shaken off any excess batter, and then dipped into the remaining breadcrumbs to coat. After evenly covered, transfer to the baking sheet with lined sides. When necessary, work in batches, and add extra bread crumbs if they start to get clumpy and soggy.
- To ensure that each cauliflower floret gets crispy, place the cauliflower in a single layer on the baking sheet, leaving space between them. If necessary, use two baking sheets.
- Brush the cauliflower with avocado oil and bake it for twenty to twenty-five minutes, rotating it halfway through, or until it is crispy and browned on all sides.
- In the meantime, combine spicy sauce, maple syrup, coconut oil, and garlic powder to make buffalo sauce.
- Remove the crispy cauliflower wings from the oven and coat them with buffalo sauce, either by brushing it on or drizzling it on. After baking for an additional five to ten minutes, or until the crust reaches the desired level of crispness, serve with our Yogurt Ranch Dip and carrot and celery sticks.

Nutritional Facts: Calories 310kcal, Fat 18g, Carbohydrates 33g, Protein 6g, Sodium 386mg, Calcium 109mg. Phosphorus mg, Potassium 423mg

73. Vegetable and Tofu Stir-Fry

Cooking time: 54 mins   **Yield:** 4

Ingredients

- One cup of long-grain rice
- A half-tbsp of hoisin sauce
- Double-tablet lime juice
- One 454g container of medium-firm tofu that has been treated with calcium sulfate and sliced into 1/2-inch cubes
- One tablespoon of canola oil
- One carrot, thinly sliced
- One bell pepper, cut thinly
- 1 teaspoon freshly grated ginger
- Two cups of bean sprouts
- four thinly cut scallions
- two tablespoons finely chopped, roasted peanuts
- 1/4 cup of raw cilantro

Instructions

- Get the rice cooked.
- Mix lime juice and hoisin sauce together.
- In a large skillet, heat the oil over medium-high heat. Stir-fry the carrot, bell pepper, and ginger for two minutes after adding them. Add the bean sprouts and tofu. Stir-fry for 3 to 4 minutes, or until the vegetables are just starting to soften. It is crucial that the bean sprouts are cooked through for food safety.
- Serve the vegetables over rice after tossing them with the hoisin sauce combination.
- If preferred, add a sprinkle of cilantro, peanuts, and scallions.
- Be aware that certain varieties of Hoisin sauce include a potassium preservative in the ingredient list; select one without!

Nutritional Facts: Calories 319kcal, Fat 12g, Carbohydrates 39g, Protein 19g, Sodium 175mg, Phosphorus 196mg, Potassium 382mg

74. Garlic Mashed Potatoes

Cooking time: 30 mins   **Yield:** 4

Ingredients

- two medium-sized potatoes
- two cloves of garlic
- 1/4 cup of butter
- 1/4 cup One percent low-fat milk

Instructions

- Potatoes should be peeled and cut into small pieces. If you follow a low-potassium diet, double-boil to lower the potassium content.
- Add the garlic and potatoes to a medium-high boil until tender.

- Remove the cooking water by draining.
- Using a mixer, blend potatoes and garlic until smooth, then gradually add butter and milk.

Nutritional Facts: Calories 185kcal, Fat 13g, Carbohydrates 15g, Protein 2g, Sodium 103mg, Calcium 35mg. Phosphorus 65mg, Potassium 205mg

75. BAKED TILAPIA FILETS GREMOLATA

Cooking time: 40 mins   **Yield:** 4

Ingredients

- Baked Tilapia
- Four skinless tilapia fillets (6 oz apiece)
- Gremolata
- One cup of parsley
- 2 tsp finely grated lemon zest
- Four to six garlic cloves

Instructions

- In a food processor, pulse all the ingredients together to make the gremolata.
- Regarding the tilapia: Set oven temperature to 375°F.
- The filets should be seasoned with black pepper and placed on a baking sheet.

- Distribute the gremolata evenly over the fish.
- Bake the fish for about 15 minutes, or until it's opaque throughout.

Nutritional Facts: Calories 202kcal, Fat 3g, Carbohydrates 2g, Protein 41g, Sodium 114mg, Phosphorus 354mg, Potassium 705mg

76. QUINOA DRESSING

Cooking time: 40 mins   **Yield:** 6

Ingredients

- One cup of onions
- two cups of celery
- 1 cup of vegetable stock low in salt
- one cup of water
- 3/4 cup of raw quinoa
- 1/4 cup of butter without salt
- Two tsp of desiccated parsley
- One tablespoon of dried sage
- half a teaspoon of powdered garlic
- half a teaspoon of black pepper, ground
- Dried cranberries, half a cup

Instructions

- Set oven temperature to 350° F.
- Dice celery and chop onion. Put aside.
- In a medium saucepan, combine the water and stock; heat to a boil. Return to a boil after adding the quinoa and

stirring. The quinoa should absorb all of the liquid after 12 minutes of simmering, covered, and low heat.

- Meanwhile, heat a large skillet over medium heat to melt butter. After about ten minutes, or until the onion and celery are transparent, toss in them and stir occasionally.
- Take the onion mixture off of the burner. To the onion mixture, add the quinoa. Add the pepper, garlic, sage, and parsley and stir. Stir well.
- Mix the cranberries into the dressing.
- After transferring the dressing to an 8" square pan, bake it for half an hour.

Nutritional Facts: Calories 205kcal, Fat 9g, Carbohydrates 27g, Protein 4g, Sodium mg, Calcium 50mg. Phosphorus 132mg, Potassium 297mg

77. GRILLED MARINATED CHICKEN

Cooking time: 40 mins   **Yield:** 4

Ingredients

- Four skinless and boneless chicken breasts
- One clove of garlic
- one-fourth cup olive oil
- One-fourth cup red wine vinegar
- One tsp powdered onion

- 1.5 tsp of dry combination of Italian seasoning
- Half a teaspoon of fresh or dried thyme sprigs (optional)

Instructions

- Cut the chicken breasts in half lengthwise, resulting in two slender filets each breast.
- Finely chop the garlic and put it in a zip-top bag with the other ingredients. Give everything a good stir.
- To the bag, add the chicken filets. Close the lid and let the food marinade for at least two hours, rotating it now and again.
- After removing the chicken from the marinade, cook it for about 10 minutes on medium heat, flipping it once. A meat thermometer should read 165 degrees Fahrenheit. If desired, garnish the chicken while it's grilling with fresh thyme sprigs.

Nutritional Facts: Calories 265kcal, Fat 17g, Carbohydrates 1g, Protein 27g, Sodium 65mg, Calcium 31mg. Phosphorus 200mg, Potassium 252mg

78. SPINACH AND FETA STUFFED CHICKEN BREAST

Cooking time: 40 mins   **Yield:** 8

Ingredients

- One pound of thin shoots of asparagus
- Eight ounces of skin-and bone-free chicken breasts
- 16 ounces of raw penne noodles
- Five tsp of olive oil
- 1/4 tsp black pepper
- one-fourth teaspoon powdered garlic
- Half a cup of chicken broth with minimal sodium
- One clove of garlic
- one and a half tsp dried oregano
- 1/4 cup of feta cheese, crumbled

Instructions

- Trim asparagus and cut into 1-inch slices on the diagonal. Cube up the chicken.
- Heat up a big saucepan of water until it boils. Add the pasta and cook for 8 to 10 minutes, or as directed on the package. Don't season with salt. After draining, put aside.
- In a large skillet, warm up 3 tablespoons of olive oil over medium-high heat. Add the chicken and season with garlic powder and pepper. Cook for about 5 minutes, or until chicken is cooked through and browned. Transfer the chicken to paper towels.
- Fill the skillet with the chicken broth. Add the chopped garlic, asparagus, oregano, pepper, and a tsp more of the garlic powder.

- For about five minutes, or until the asparagus is barely tender, cover and steam.
- Place the chicken back in the skillet and reheat it well.
- Mix thoroughly after adding the chicken stuff to the noodles. Give it a five-minute wait.
- After another toss, drizzle with the remaining two tablespoons of olive oil and top with feta cheese.

Nutritional Facts: Calories 376kcal, Fat 12g, Carbohydrates 49g, Protein 18g, Sodium 110mg, Calcium 58mg. Phosphorus 193mg, Potassium 243mg

79. LINGUINE WITH GARLIC AND SHRIMP

Cooking time: 25 mins   **Yield:** 6

Ingredients

- three-quarter pound of raw shrimp
- One cup parsley, flat-leaf
- two and a half pints of water
- 12 ounces of raw linguine
- Two tsp olive oil
- two entire heads of garlic
- One tablespoon of lemon juice
- 1/4 tsp black pepper

Instructions

- Clean and peel the shrimp. Finely chop the parsley.
- Fill a big pot with boiling water. When the pasta is tender, add it and simmer for ten minutes.
- Peel and divide the garlic cloves as the pasta cooks. In a frying pan, toast the cloves over medium heat, turning constantly. When the garlic turns dark and becomes tender to the touch, it is ready. It will be simple to remove skin. Peel the garlic's skin and remove it from the pan.
- Return the peeled garlic to the frying pan and add some heated olive oil. Sauté the garlic until it turns golden. (Cloves can be divided in half or not.)
- Once the shrimp turns pink, simmer for one to two minutes after adding the parsley.
- After draining, set aside one cup of the liquid. Put spaghetti, garlic, and shrimp in a pan. Combine all ingredients and stir in the cup of liquid that was set aside.
- Add the black pepper and lemon juice. Blend and proceed to serve.

Nutritional Facts: Calories 322kcal, Fat 6g, Carbohydrates 47g, Protein 20g, Sodium 106mg, Calcium 87mg. Phosphorus 220mg, Potassium 298mg

80. VEGETABLE LENTIL SOUP

Cooking time: 35 mins   **Yield:** 4

Ingredients

- One tsp extra virgin olive oil
- chopped celery stalks
- chopped carrots
- diced sweet onion
- ½ cup of lentils
- Five cups of low-sodium chicken stock or broth
- Two cups of thinly sliced chard leaves
- freshly ground black pepper, to taste
- One lemon's juice

Instructions

- Heat the olive oil in a medium stockpot over medium-high heat. Stir the onion for three to five minutes, or until it becomes tender.
- Stir in the lentils, celery, carrots, and broth. After bringing to a boil, lower the heat, and simmer the lentils for 15 minutes without a lid until they become soft.
- After adding the shard, simmer for a further three minutes, or until it wilts.
- Add the lemon juice and pepper for seasoning. Serve.

Nutritional Facts: Calories 190kcal, Fat 6g, Carbohydrates 25g, Protein 11g, Sodium 198mg, Calcium 53mg. Phosphorus 139mg, Potassium 468mg

81. ROASTED ASPARAGUS AND WILD MUSHROOM STEW

Cooking time: 1hr 15 mins   **Yield:** 1

Ingredients

- 1 pound asparagus.
- 1 ounce of dried wild mushroom medley.
- 1 cup of very hot water.
- 2 teaspoons olive oil
- Two celery stalks.
- One carrot stick.
- 1 tiny onion.
- 1 fennel (anise) head,
- 4 fresh thyme sprigs
- pinch cayenne pepper
- ground black pepper to taste.
- 1 teaspoon of dried sage.
- 1 tablespoon of fresh, chopped parsley
- 1 tablespoon and 1 teaspoon dry Marsala wine
- 1 bay leaf and ⅛ teaspoon garlic powder.
- ⅛ teaspoon onion powder.
- 2 cups vegetable stock with low sodium.
- 2 ounces of pine nuts.

Instructions

- Preheat the oven to 400°F. Wash and trim the rough bottoms of asparagus spears.
- Arrange the asparagus stalks in a single layer on a baking sheet. Spray the spears with olive oil. (1 teaspoon of olive oil poured onto spears) Bake in the oven for ten minutes. Allow the spears to cool before cutting into 1-inch sections.
- Rehydrate dried mushrooms in 1 cup of very hot water.
- In a nonstick sauce pan, heat 1 teaspoon olive oil over medium-high heat. Add diced celery, carrots, onions, and fennel and sauté until the onions are translucent. Stir in the thyme, cayenne pepper, sage, chopped parsley, Marsala wine, bay leaf, garlic powder, and onion powder, and cook for another minute over medium heat. Simmer for 15 minutes with vegetable stock, dried mushroom liquid, and sliced wild mushrooms.
- Place the asparagus on the plate, then pour the stew and sprinkle it with pine nuts before serving.

Nutritional Facts: Calories 103kcal, Fat 5.8g, Carbohydrates 11.8g, Protein 3.4g, Sodium 78.8mg, Calcium 45.9mg, Phosphorus 60.8mg, Potassium 436.8mg

82. CHICKPEA CAULIFLOWER CURRY

Cooking time: 30 mins   **Yield:** 6

Ingredients

- One medium cauliflower head
- One fifteen-ounce can of chickpeas
- Two tablespoons of curry powder
- One medium-sized onion, either yellow or white
- one garlic clove
- One teaspoon finely chopped ginger
- One liter, or four cups vegetable broth with no additional salt
- ¼ cup coconut milk in cans (Tip: save remaining can for later by freezing in ice cube trays or reusable containers.)
- 2 Tbsp finely chopped cilantro
- One and a half cups of raw white rice

Instructions

- Use your preferred technique to cook the rice in a rice cooker or on the stovetop (for instance, put the rice in a small pot with three cups of water and bring it to a boil, then cover and cook for twenty minutes on low heat). Use a fork to fluff.
- Dice the garlic and onion.
- Cut the cauliflower into small pieces or chop it.
- Pot should be heated to medium heat. When the saucepan is heated, add the oil and the onions. Cook for three to five minutes.
- Stir for a minute after adding the ginger and curry powder.
- Add the veggie stock and the cauliflower florets. After bringing to a boil, simmer for ten minutes.
- After the chickpeas have been rinsed and drained, return them to the pot and boil again for five minutes, or until the cauliflower is soft.
- Take off the heat and stir in the coconut milk.
- Garnish with cilantro and serve with rice. Serve with butter and naan bread, if desired.

Nutritional Facts: Calories 381kcal, Fat 9g, Carbohydrates 64g, Protein 11g, Sodium 444mg, Phosphorus 180mg, Potassium 576mg

83. GRILLED VEGETABLES

Cooking time: 1hr 5mins   **Yield:** ½ cup

Ingredients

- Three medium zucchinis, sliced
- two sliced anise (fennel) heads
- eight button mushrooms, and quartered
- Cut four Roma tomatoes into eighths.
- One red onion, sliced after being cut in half
- Two tablespoons of freshly shredded basil
- 1 tsp of new thyme
- one-tsp of new oregano

Instructions

- Cut the tomatoes into eight pieces, slice the onion, chop the fennel, slice the zucchini, shred the basil leaves, and sprinkle with oregano and thyme.
- Combine all of the vegetables in a large bowl.
- Grilling outside: Oil a grill basket to fry the veggies in and set it on the preheating grill while your grill preheats to 400° F.
- Once the basket is heated, transfer your mixture of vegetables inside and cook until the vegetables take on a golden-brown color. To ensure that all of the vegetables brown evenly, don't forget to stir them every five to seven minutes.
- Broil: Press the broil button on your oven. Arrange the vegetables on a cookie sheet in a single layer, then broil until the vegetables start to take on a golden-brown hue. Vegetables should be turned over and continued to broil until soft.

Nutritional Facts: Calories 108kcal, Fat 1.1g, Carbohydrates 23.8g, Protein 5.5g, Sodium 68.9mg, Calcium 124.6mg. Phosphorus 82.6mg, Potassium 1324.1mg

84. CRUNCHY TOFU STIR FRY

Cooking time: 30 mins   **Yield:** 4

Ingredients

- sixteen ounces of extra firm tofu
- half a red bell pepper
- One clove of garlic
- 1-1/2 tablespoons of soy sauce with lower sodium
- one and a half tablespoons lime juice
- Two tablespoons cornstarch
- two teaspoons sugar
- two white eggs
- Half a cup of plain bread crumbs
- A half-tsp canola oil
- One tablespoon of sesame oil
- Fresh broccoli florets, one cup
- One tsp Mrs. Dash® herb spice blend
- one-eighth teaspoon of black pepper
- one-eighth teaspoon of cayenne
- one-half teaspoon of sesame seeds
- Two cups of white rice, steamed

Instructions

- Cube up the tofu. Slice the bell pepper and finely cut the clove of garlic.
- In a small bowl, combine sugar, lime juice, and reduced-sodium soy sauce. Put aside.
- Place the bread crumbs, egg whites, and cornstarch in three different bowls. Tofu cubes are dipped in egg whites, then cornstarch, and finally bread crumbs.
- Coated tofu is stir-fried in hot canola oil in a skillet or wok until it turns

golden brown and crisps. Take out the tofu and place it aside.

- Heat the sesame oil in the same pan. Crisp-tender broccoli and slices of red bell pepper are stir-fried. Cook for one minute after adding the minced garlic, cayenne pepper, black pepper, and Mrs. Dash seasoning blend.
- Return the tofu to the pan and mix it with the veggies. Overtop, drizzle the soy-lime juice combination, add sesame seeds, and stir. Take off the heat and split into four pieces. Accompany with half a cup of rice.

Nutritional Facts: Calories 400kcal, Fat 16g, Carbohydrates 45g, Protein 19g, Sodium 584mg, Calcium 253mg. Phosphorus 177mg, Potassium 317mg

85. EGGPLANT PARMIGIANA

Cooking time: 35 mins   **Yield:** 2

Ingredients

- One eggplant 40 g breadsticks devoid of protein
- 200 grams of tomato sauce
- 250 milliliters of seed oil
- 40 grams of cheese Parmigiano Reggiano
- Five basil leaves

Instructions

- Slice the eggplant thinly, then blanch it for 30 seconds in boiling, unsalted water. This process should be repeated twice more.
- The eggplant slices should then be dried using absorbent paper.
- Place the eggplant slices in a skillet with heating oil and fry them.
- Partially coat the bottom of a skillet with tomato sauce, then put a layer of eggplant slices over the whole thing.
- Next, add another layer of tomato sauce, followed by a scattering of crushed protein-free breadsticks and basil leaves.
- Until you run out of ingredients, keep adding layers.
- Lastly, bake for 10 minutes at 180° in the oven.

Nutritional Facts: Calories 334kcal, Fat 28g, Protein 2g, Sodium 37mg, Phosphorus 67mg, Potassium 306mg

86. SHRIMP-STUFFED DEVILED EGGS

Cooking time: 30 mins   **Yield:** 6

Ingredients

- Six big hard-boiled eggs
- half a cup of cooked shrimp
- half a teaspoon of mustard
- One and a half tablespoons of mayo

- half a teaspoon of lemon juice
- 1/4 tsp black pepper

Instructions

- Halve cooked eggs lengthwise. Remove yolks with care, then transfer to a bowl.
- Chop the shrimp finely, then mix the egg yolks with the mustard, mayonnaise, lemon juice, and pepper. Stir until all of the ingredients are incorporated.
- Pile the shrimp and yolk mixture into the halves of egg whites.

Nutritional Facts: Calories 112kcal, Fat 8g, Carbohydrates 1g, Protein 9g, Sodium 113mg, Calcium 33mg. Phosphorus 122mg, Potassium 93mg

87. HERB PESTO TUNA

Cooking time: 20 mins   **Yield:** 4

Ingredients

- Four (three-ounce) filets of yellowfin tuna
- One tsp olive oil
- A half-cup of herb pesto
- freshly ground black pepper, to taste
- 1 lemon, thinly sliced into 8 pieces

Instructions

- Preheat the grill to medium-high heat.

- After drizzling the fish with olive oil, sprinkle pepper on each filet.
- Grill the fish for four minutes on a grill.
- After flipping the fish, place lemon slices and the herb pesto on top of each piece.
- Cook the tuna for a further 5 to 6 minutes, or until it reaches a medium-well doneness.

Nutritional Facts: Calories 121kcal, Fat 3g, Carbohydrates 0g, Protein 21g, Sodium 38mg, Calcium 8mg. Phosphorus 238mg, Potassium 386mg

88. VEGETABLE CURRY

Cooking time: 60 mins   **Yield:** 5

Ingredients

- One teaspoon each of cumin, coriander, and mustard seeds
- one-half teaspoon of black peppercorns
- one-teaspoon of fennel seeds
- one teaspoon of coriander seeds
- Two cups of basmati rice
- One tablespoon of coconut oil
- One 2-inch piece of finely grated ginger
- One tsp of turmeric
- ½ teaspoon of spicy chili powder
- One medium (70g) chopped onion

- one can of coconut milk
- One cup of frozen green peas
- One medium (61g) sliced carrot
- 1½ cups of bite-sized cauliflower florets

Instructions

- In a cast-iron skillet, warm the dry spices for two minutes over low to medium heat.
- As the spices heat, prepare the rice according to the package's instructions.
- Add the coconut oil and sauté for two to three minutes, or until the spices are popping and lightly browned.
- Stir in the turmeric, ginger, and hot chili flakes. Simmer for six minutes on low to medium heat, or until fragrant.
- Take off the heat and put the cooked spices and onion in a blender to make a paste.
- Heat the coconut milk until it begins to bubble in a different pan. Incorporate the spice paste and blend well with a whisk.
- After preparing the veggies, add them and boil for about ten minutes, or until they are just soft.
- Enjoy a cup of curry served over rice!

Nutritional Facts: Calories 318kcal, Fat 20g, Carbohydrates 30g, Protein 6g, Sodium 33mg, Calcium 58mg. Phosphorus 175mg, Potassium 477mg

89. SUMMER GARDEN EGGPLANT

Cooking time: 50 mins   **Yield:** 4

Ingredients

- three cups of eggplant
- One tablespoon each of onion, celery, and parsley
- one-fourth cup bell pepper, green
- one-fourth cup red bell pepper
- Half a tablespoon of unsalted butter
- One tsp Mrs. Dash® herb and onion seasoning
- One cup of moist bread crumbs

Instructions

- Set oven temperature to 350° F.
- Dice the eggplant into half-inch chunks. For the recipe, measure three cups. Chop the bell peppers, celery, onion, and parsley.
- Combine the vegetables.
- Apply cooking spray to a 1-1/2-quart baking dish. Cover after adding the vegetable mixture. Bake for forty minutes.
- Melt the margarine and combine the soft bread crumbs with Mrs. Dash® herb spice while the vegetables bake.
- Take off the baking dish's cover and add the crumb mixture. Put the dish back in the oven, uncovered. Bake for

a further 10 minutes, or until the topping starts to softly brown.

Nutritional Facts: Calories 101kcal, Fat 6g, Carbohydrates 10g, Protein 2g, Sodium 66mg, Calcium 20mg. Phosphorus 30mg, Potassium 183mg

90. CITRUS SALMON

Cooking time: 35 mins   **Yield:** 6

Ingredients

- two cloves of garlic
- one and a half tablespoons of lemon juice
- Two tsp olive oil
- One tablespoon each of butter and Dijon mustard
- Two cayenne pepper dashes
- One tsp of dehydrated basil leaves
- One tsp of dried dill
- One tablespoon of capers
- A 24-oz salmon filet

Instructions

- Mash the garlic.
- Combine all the ingredients, excluding the salmon, in a small saucepan. Bring to a boil, then lower the heat to a simmer and cook for an additional five minutes.
- Heat the grill in the interim. Place the salmon on a piece of foil that is just a little bit bigger than the fish, skin side down. To ensure that the sauce stays with the salmon on the grill, fold up the edges. Place the fish on the grill with the foil. Drizzle the salmon with the previously made sauce.
- Once the salmon is cooked, cover the grill and cook for 12 minutes. Salmon should not be flipped. Divide the salmon into six portions.

Nutritional Facts: Calories 294kcal, Fat 22g, Carbohydrates 1g, Protein 23g, Sodium 190mg, Calcium 21mg. Phosphorus 280mg, Potassium 439mg

91. ZESTY RICE SALAD

Cooking time: 30 mins   **Yield:** 3

Ingredients

For the Dressing

- Two tsp miso paste
- Two tsp of maple syrup
- One tablespoon of olive oil
- two limes, squeezed
- one garlic clove
- Half a jalapeño, cut open
- 1 tsp apple cider vinegar

For the Salad

- Brown basmati rice, 4 ounces
- 1/2 medium (95 grams) yellow squash, quartered and sliced into rounds

- 2 oz of large (180 grams) carrots
- 2 oz of green onions, diced
- 1 tbsp sesame seeds
- Two tablespoons of ripped mint
- two tablespoons shredded cilantro

Special Gadgets

- Grater
- Blender
- Steamer Basket

Instructions

Instructions For Making The Salad Dressing

- Pour the ingredients for the dressing into a high-speed blender.
- Process till smooth.

Instructions For Making The Salad

- Follow the instructions on the package to cook the rice. Spoon into a large mixing bowl after draining.
- A medium-sized saucepan should be heated to medium-high heat. Pour in two inches of water.
- Bring to a boil, insert the squash, and cover with a steamer basket.
- After covering the squash with a lid, steam it for four minutes, or until it becomes soft.
- In a medium-sized mixing dish, combine steamed summer squash, carrots, green onions, and sesame seeds. Blend thoroughly.

- Over the salad in the mixing bowl, drizzle the dressing. Stir till the dressing coats everything.
- Transfer the salad into separate serving bowls and decorate with the cilantro and mint.

Nutritional Facts: Calories 258kcal, Fat 8g, Carbohydrates 44g, Protein 5g, Sodium 150mg, Calcium 86mg. Phosphorus 188mg, Potassium 496mg

92. SEAFOOD CASSEROLE

Cooking time: 50 mins   **Yield:** 8

Ingredients

- two medium eggplants
- One medium onion
- One bell pepper
- 1/2 cup celery
- 2 cloves of garlic
- one-fourth cup olive oil
- one-fourth cup lemon juice
- One tablespoon of Worcestershire sauce
- 1/4 tsp of seasoning for creole
- Half a teaspoon of hot sauce (Tabasco®)
- one-third cup raw rice
- One-fourth cup of Parmesan cheese
- One dash of cayenne
- Three big eggs
- One pound of flesh from lump crabs

- Half a pound of cooked shrimp
- Half a cup of bread crumbs
- Two tablespoons of melted butter

Instructions

- Turn the oven on to 350°F.
- Chop the celery, bell pepper, and onion. Dice and peel the eggplant into 1-inch pieces.
- In a medium saucepan, place the eggplant, cover with water, and boil for about five minutes, or until soft. Thoroughly drain, transfer to a mixing dish, and reserve.
- In olive oil, sauté the onion, bell pepper, celery, and garlic until they are soft but not browned.
- Incorporate sautéed veggies into the eggplant. Stir in the beaten eggs, rice, parmesan cheese, cayenne, Worcestershire sauce, Creole seasonings, and lemon juice. Mix thoroughly by stirring.
- Fold fish gently into a mixture of vegetables. Put in a casserole dish that has been oiled.
- Top casserole with melted butter and bread crumbs.
- Bake until the topping starts to brown, 25 to 30 minutes.

Nutritional Facts: Calories 216kcal, Fat 12g, Carbohydrates 14g, Protein 13g, Sodium 229mg, Calcium 79mg. Phosphorus 148mg, Potassium 359mg

93. ROTINI WITH MOCK ITALIAN SAUSAGE

Cooking time: 60 mins   **Yield:** 4

Ingredients

- Four ounces of raw rotini pasta
- Lean ground turkey, ¾ pound
- One cup chopped onion, one minced garlic clove, and one-half cup chopped celery
- One-half teaspoon of Italian spice
- ¼ tsp fennel powder
- A tsp of finely ground red pepper
- Tomato paste, three teaspoons
- One to 14 and a half unsalted can (190 grams) of chopped tomatoes
- two teaspoons of grated parmesan cheese

Instructions

- As directed on the package, boil the rotini pasta and then drain.
- In a nonstick skillet, cook the turkey over medium heat until it is browned, turning to break it up.
- Using paper towels, drain.
- Add the seasonings, celery, onion, and garlic. Cook, stirring periodically, for 3 minutes.
- Add the tomatoes and tomato paste. Lower the heat, partially cover, and simmer for fifteen minutes.

- Put on top of rotini. Add cheese on top.

Nutritional Facts: Calories 165kcal, Fat 0g, Carbohydrates 28g, Protein 13g, Sodium 250mg, Calcium 65mg. Phosphorus 161mg, Potassium 458mg

94. QUICK PAN-GLAZED CHICKEN

Cooking time: 40 mins   **Yield:** 4

Ingredients

- two tsp olive oil
- One-pound chicken breasts, deboned and skinless
- 1/4 tsp black pepper
- Three tsp balsamic vinegar
- three tsp honey
- two tsp of dried basil

Instructions

- In a pan set over medium heat, warm the olive oil. Add the chicken, then season with pepper.
- Brown the chicken by sautéing it for five minutes on each side.
- After adding the balsamic vinegar, sauté the chicken for one minute, turning it over to coat.
- Add the basil and honey. To coat, stir and turn the chicken. Simmer for a further minute.

- Transfer to a platter and cover the chicken with the pan sauce.

Nutritional Facts: Calories 209kcal, Fat 5g, Carbohydrates 15g, Protein 26g, Sodium 55mg, Calcium 18mg. Phosphorus 246mg, Potassium 412mg

95. LAMB CHOPS WITH REDCURRANT & MINT SAUCE

Cooking time: 50 mins   **Yield:** 4

Ingredients

- 4 x 140g or 5 ½ ounce, fat-trimmed lamb chops
- 1/2 lemon juice
- 4 tbsp redcurrant jelly
- 4 tablespoons of Water
- 1 heaping tablespoon of cornflour (approx.)

Instructions

- Combine red currant jelly, mint sauce, lemon juice, and water in a casserole dish that may be baked in the oven.
- After trimming, add chops to mixture and turn to coat.
- The lamb should be baked uncovered for 30 to 45 minutes at 180 degrees Celsius / Gas Mark 4 until it is tender.
- Before serving, use the cornflour and a small amount of water to thicken the sauce.

Nutritional Facts: Calories 216kcal, Fat 7.8g, Carbohydrates 15g, Protein 23g, Sodium 300mg, Phosphorus 218mg, Potassium 10mmol

96. FISH TACOS

Cooking time: 55 mins　　　　**Yield:** 6

Ingredients

- 1-1/2 cups of cabbage
- Half a cup red onion
- half a handful of cilantros
- One clove of garlic
- two limes
- One-pound filets of cod
- half a teaspoon of cumin powder
- Half a teaspoon of red pepper flakes
- 1/4 tsp black pepper
- One tablespoon of olive oil
- one-half cup mayonnaise
- One-fourth cup sour cream
- two tsp milk
- 12 six-inch corn tortillas

Instructions

- Chop the cilantro, onion, and cabbage, and shred it. Put aside. Dice the garlic.
- Squeeze the juice of 1/2 a lime over the fish fillets that have been placed on a platter. Add olive oil, chili powder, cumin, black pepper, and minced garlic to the filets. After turning the filets to coat them with marinade, chill them for a half hour or more.
- Combine mayonnaise, sour cream, milk, and half a lime juice to make salsa blanca. After combining, put in the fridge to cool.
- Preheat the oven to broil. Use foil to cover the broiler pan. Fish should be broiled for about ten minutes, or until the flesh turns opaque and white and the fish flakes readily. Take the fish out of the oven, let it cool a little, and then break it into big pieces.
- One by one, reheat the corn tortillas in a pan until they are tender and warm. To keep them warm, cover them with a fresh dish towel.
- Tacos are assembled by placing a piece of fish on a tortilla, then adding cabbage, red onion, cilantro, and lime wedges on top. If you want, add hot sauce.

Nutritional Facts: Calories 363kcal, Fat 19g, Carbohydrates 30g, Protein 18g, Sodium 194mg, Calcium 138mg. Phosphorus 327mg, Potassium 507mg

97. COUSCOUS WITH VEGETABLES

Cooking time: 20 mins　　　　**Yield:** 5

Ingredients

- One spoonful of margarine
- half a cup of frozen peas
- A quarter cup of raw mushrooms
- 1/2 cup onion
- One clove of garlic
- two tsp of dry white wine
- half a teaspoon of dried basil
- one-eighth teaspoon of black pepper
- Two tsp of raw parsley
- Half a cup of uncooked couscous

Instructions

- Defrost the peas outside. Slice the mushrooms thinly, mince the onion, and crush the garlic. Chop the parsley.
- Melt the margarine in a nonstick pan.
- Add the wine, peas, onion, and mushrooms. Stirring often, sauté for 5 minutes.
- Blend thoroughly after adding the spices. Stir in parsley well. Take off the heat and place aside.
- Follow the Instructions on the package to prepare the couscous.
- Combine the prepared couscous and veggie mixture in a large bowl. Serve right away.

Nutritional Facts: Calories 104kcal, Fat 2g, Carbohydrates 18g, Protein 3g, Sodium 33mg, Calcium 18mg. Phosphorus 52mg, Potassium 100mg

98. SPANISH RICE

Cooking time: 20 mins   **Yield:** 6

Ingredients

- half a cup of onions
- half a cup of pepper, green
- One tablespoon of olive oil
- One cup raw rice
- one tsp powdered garlic
- Half a teaspoon of red pepper flakes
- 1/4 cup tomato puree with low sodium
- two cups of water

Instructions

- Dice the green pepper and onion.
- Heat a skillet with olive oil and sauté onions and green pepper until they become tender.
- When the rice begins to softly brown, add it to the skillet and stir continuously.
- To the skillet, add the tomato puree, chili powder, garlic powder, and water. For about 15 to 20 minutes, or until the rice is soft and the water has been absorbed, cover and simmer over low heat.

Nutritional Facts: Calories 134kcal, Fat 3g, Carbohydrates 25g, Protein 1g, Sodium 7mg, Calcium 7mg. Phosphorus 53mg, Potassium 139mg

99. GOURMET GREEN BEANS

Cooking time: 40 mins   **Yield:** 4

Ingredients

- Frozen green beans, 10 ounces
- Four tsp margarine
- one-fourth cup onion
- Half a cup of red bell pepper
- One tsp of dried dill
- One tsp of dehydrated parsley
- 1/4 tsp black pepper

Instructions

- Boil the green beans until they are soft. Empty.
- Dice the bell pepper and onion.
- Put a skillet over medium heat, add margarine, and cook the onion, red pepper, parsley, and dill until they are tender.
- After adding the green beans to the skillet, cook them through.
- After adding a dash of black pepper, serve.

Nutritional Facts: Calories 67kcal, Fat 3g, Carbohydrates 8g, Protein 2g, Sodium 55mg, Calcium 68mg. Phosphorus 32mg, Potassium 194mg

100.   KIDNEY BEAN SALAD

Cooking time: 10 mins   **Yield:** 6

Ingredients

For the salad

- One and a half cups (1 x 15 oz can) of kidney beans, drained and rinsed
- One and a half cups (1 x 15 oz can) of washed, drained, and mashed chickpeas
- One medium-sized sliced cucumber
- one medium-sized finely chopped sweet white or red onion
- One cup, or two large handfuls of parsley leaves, flat, cut or torn

Regarding the dressing

- Five tsp freshly squeezed lemon juice, roughly one large juicy lemon or one and a half medium ones
- Three tablespoons of extra virgin olive oil (omit if you want to make it oil-free)
- Two tiny garlic cloves, finely chopped or grated
- One to two tsp sugar, or a tiny drop of agave or maple syrup
- 1/2 tsp salt, or to taste 1/2 tsp freshly ground black pepper, or to taste

Instructions

- Place the beans in a big salad bowl after draining and rinsing.
- Add the chopped onion, parsley, and cucumber.

- Mix all the dressing ingredients together with a whisk or shake well in a container. To achieve the ideal ratio of sweet to tangy for you, I advise increasing the sugar to taste.
- Drizzle the salad with the dressing and mix well.

Nutritional Facts: Calories 205kcal, Fat 8g, Carbohydrates 26g, Protein 8g, Sodium 200mg, Calcium 44mg, Potassium 381mg

CHAPTER 7

MEAT & POULTRY RECIPES

101. BARLEY RICE

Cooking time: 60 mins   **Yield**: 4

Ingredients

- ⅓ cup dried pearled barley
- One-third cup dry short-grain white rice
- One tablespoon of butter without salt
- 1/2 cup chopped celery
- 1/2 cup chopped carrots
- 1/2 cup chopped red onion
- 2 ¼ cups unsalted chicken broth
- A single tsp of dried thyme
- One tsp poultry seasoning

Instructions

- Wash the rice and barley in cold water until the water runs clear. Put aside.
- Melt the butter in a pot over a medium heat. Add the celery, carrots, and onions until heated through. Simmer onions for 45 minutes, or until they are tender.
- Stir continuously for 1 minute after adding the rice and barley.
- Stir in the poultry seasoning, thyme, and chicken broth. Heat till boiling.
- Once the liquid has been absorbed, reduce heat to a simmer, cover, and cook for 35 minutes.
- Take off the heat source, take off the cover, and cover with a cloth. Give it ten minutes to rest.
- Using a fork, fluff after resting.

Nutritional Facts: Calories 184kcal, Fat 4g, Carbohydrates 32g, Protein 6g, Sodium 98mg, Calcium 35mg. Phosphorus 110mg, Potassium 299mg

102. CHICKEN AND SUMMER VEGETABLE KEBABS

Cooking time: 45 mins   **Yield:** 4

Ingredients

- A tsp of peach jam
- Two tsp olive oil
- two tsp lemon juice
- One tsp Mrs. Dash® herb spice blend
- 1/4 tsp salt
- One-pound chicken thighs, deboned and skinless
- One medium zucchini
- One medium yellow summer squash
- One red bell pepper
- One medium onion

Instructions

- Measure the peach jam into a small microwave-safe bowl and liquefy it for 10 to 15 seconds to make the marinade. Add the lemon juice, salt, Mrs. Dash® herb spice, and olive oil. Blend thoroughly by stirring.
- After rinsing, use paper towels to pat the chicken thighs dry. Each thigh should be cut into four pieces and put in a zip-top bag.
- Toss the chicken pieces with 3 tablespoons of marinade. (Save two tablespoons of the marinade for veggies.) Let the bag marinate in the refrigerator after sealing it.
- For the kebabs, chop the veggies (onion varies), red pepper into sixteen pieces, zucchini into eight slices, and yellow squash into eight slices. Add the marinade that was set aside to a medium-sized bowl. Coat the vegetable pieces by stirring.
- Put the chicken pieces and veggies onto 4 big or 8 little skewers.
- Turn the grill's heat to medium. After putting the skewers on the grill, cover and cook for 12 to 15 minutes. For even cooking, turn the skewers two or three times.

Nutritional Facts: Calories 284kcal, Fat 16g, Carbohydrates 10g, Protein 24g, Sodium 215mg, Calcium 30mg. Phosphorus 194mg, Potassium 456mg

103.   INDIAN CHICKEN CURRY

Cooking time: 60 mins   **Yield:** 6

Ingredients

- One medium-sized tomato
- two medium-sized onions
- two cloves of garlic
- One inch square piece of ginger root
- Five tsp vegetable oil
- three-quarters teaspoon of whole cumin seeds
- One cinnamon stick
- two bay leaves
- One-fourth teaspoon of whole peppercorns
- 1.5 pounds of little drumsticks made of chicken
- three-quarters teaspoon of salt
- 1-1/2 tsp cayenne pepper (or half a tsp for milder flavor)
- Half a teaspoon of garam masala

Instructions

- Chop and peel the tomato. Mince the ginger root, onion, and garlic. Take off and dispose of the chicken's skin.
- In a large, wide pot, heat the oil over medium-high heat. Add the peppercorns, bay leaves, cinnamon,

and cumin seeds when they're hot. Once, stir.

- Add the ginger, garlic, and onions. Stir this mixture until brown flecks appear on the onion.
- Add the chicken, tomatoes, cayenne, and salt. After mixing well, come to a boil.
- Once the chicken is cooked, simmer it for 25 minutes on low heat with a tight lid on the pot. Throughout this cooking time, stir a couple times.
- After removing the cover, increase the heat to medium. Add the garam masala and cook, stirring occasionally, until the liquid is reduced, about 5 minutes.

Nutritional Facts: Calories 269kcal, Fat 18g, Carbohydrates 6g, Protein 21g, Sodium 350mg, Calcium 27mg. Phosphorus 139mg, Potassium 286mg

104. CHICKEN STIR FRY

Cooking time: 40 mins   **Yield:** 6

Ingredients

- A 12-oz chicken breast that is skinless and boneless
- three tsp honey
- three teaspoons of vinegar
- three tsp pineapple juice
- 1-1/2 tablespoons of soy sauce with lower sodium
- one and a half teaspoons cornstarch
- Two tsp of canola oil
- Three cups of assorted frozen vegetables
- Three cups of freshly cooked, heated rice

Instructions

- Slice the chicken into 1-inch chunks and save.
- Combine the honey, vinegar, pineapple juice, soy sauce, and cornstarch to create the sauce and set it aside.
- Transfer canola oil onto a big wok or skillet. (If additional oil is needed when cooking.) Turn the heat up to medium-high.
- Frozen veggies should be stir-fried for three minutes, or until they become crisp-tender.
- Take out the veggies from the skillet.
- To a heated skillet, add the chicken. Stir-fry until the chicken is no longer pink, about 3 to 4 minutes. Displace the chicken from the skillet's center. Add sauce and stir; transfer to skillet's center. Cook, stirring, until bubbling and thickened.
- Place the cooked veggies back in the skillet. To coat, combine all ingredients and stir. Cook and stir for an additional minute or until well heated.
- Serve right away with rice.

Nutritional Facts: Calories 279kcal, Fat 6g, Carbohydrates 38g, Protein 17g, Sodium 196mg, Calcium 52mg. Phosphorus 180mg, Potassium 349mg

105. ALL AMERICAN MEATLOAF

Cooking time: 1hr 25mins   **Yield:** 6

Ingredients

- two tablespoons of onion
- Twenty squares of unsalted top saltine-style crackers
- One pound of 10% fat, lean ground beef
- One big egg
- two tsp One percent skim milk
- 1/4 tsp black pepper
- one-third cup catsup
- One-third cup brown sugar
- One-half tsp apple cider vinegar
- one tsp water

Instructions

- Set oven temperature to 350°F.
- Chop the onion finely. Crush the crackers with a rolling pin after placing them in a big zip-top bag.
- Apply nonstick cooking spray to a loaf pan.
- Crushed crackers, onion, ground beef, egg, milk, and black pepper should all be combined in a big bowl. Blend thoroughly.
- Fill the loaf pan with mixture. Bake for forty minutes.
- In a separate bowl, combine catsup, brown sugar, vinegar, and water to form the topping.
- Take the cooked meatloaf out of the oven and pour sauce over it.
- After 10 minutes, or until the interior temperature reaches 160° F, return the pan to the oven.
- Cut into six pieces and present.

Nutritional Facts: Calories 205kcal, Fat 9g, Carbohydrates 14g, Protein 17g, Sodium 263mg, Calcium 36mg. Phosphorus 147mg, Potassium 254mg

106. BASIL CHICKEN

Cooking time: 25 mins   **Yield:** 4

Ingredients

- Four skinless chicken breasts
- 1/3 cup of margarine without trans fat
- one-fourth cup of fresh basil
- One tbsp of finely grated Parmesan cheese
- one-fourth teaspoon of powdered garlic
- Mrs. Dash® herb seasoning combination, 1/4 teaspoon

- Four new sprigs of basil, optional garnish

Instructions

- Warm up the oven to 325°F.
- Put the halves of chicken breasts in a glass baking pan. To allow the mixture to season and flavor the breasts while they cook, pierce each one several times with a fork.
- In a glass mixing bowl, melt margarine in the microwave. Stir to disperse heat starting at 15 seconds.
- Add Mrs. Dash®, garlic powder, basil, and parmesan cheese to melted margarine. Whisk or use a fork to stir the mixture.
- Over the chicken breasts, divide the parmesan cheese evenly by pouring the mixture over them.
- Baked uncovered, basting every 10 minutes with mixture from the pan, for a total of about 25 minutes or until juices in chicken are clear, not pink.

Nutritional Facts: Calories 252kcal, Fat 16g, Carbohydrates 0g, Protein 27g, Sodium 232mg, Calcium 31mg. Phosphorus 210mg, Potassium 246mg

107. CHICKEN STUFFED AVOCADO

Cooking time: 45 mins   **Yield:** 1

Ingredients

- One tablespoon of cilantro
- Three ounces of chicken, either homemade or from a rotisserie
- Three cherry tomatoes
- One spoonful of goat cheese
- half an avocado

Instructions

- Halve a ripe avocado and transfer the contents to a bowl. You will use the shell for serving, so save it.
- A store-bought rotisserie chicken works beautifully for this. Add 3 ounces of cooked chicken and combine with avocado.
- Add three cherry tomatoes and chop them up.
- Reassemble the mixture in the avocado shell that is empty.
- Add some cilantro and goat cheese on top.

Nutritional Facts: Calories 381kcal, Fat 30g, Carbohydrates 10g, Protein 20g, Sodium 121mg

108. CRISPY SESAME CHICKEN

Cooking time: 40 mins   **Yield:** 1

Ingredients

- One tablespoon of roasted sesame seeds
- two tsp finely chopped ginger
- One tablespoon of reduced-sodium soy sauce
- two tablespoons of honey
- One tablespoon of sherry
- Four four-oz halves of peeled and boned chicken breast
- Cooking spray with vegetables

Instructions

- In a small bowl, combine the first five ingredients.
- Put aside.
- Using a rolling pin or mallet, flatten the chicken pieces to a thickness of ¼ inch.
- Apply cooking spray to the grill.
- Grill chicken over medium–hot coals 4 minutes each side, basting regularly with soy sauce mixture.
- Move the mixture to a serving dish.

Nutritional Facts: Calories 257kcal, Fat 6.5g, Carbohydrates 10g, Protein 37.8g, Sodium 237.3mg, Calcium 22.9mg. Phosphorus 282.4mg, Potassium 331.7mg

109. CHICKEN LASAGNE WITH WHITE SAUCE

Cooking time: 1hr 25mins   **Yield:** 6

Ingredients

- Six ounces of chicken (thighs or breasts)
- Low-sodium chicken broth, 12 ounces
- one-fourth cup olive oil
- one large onion, chopped
- One tablespoon of oregano
- 1/4 tsp black pepper
- 1/4 cup white wine, if desired
- Half a cup of thickly sliced mushrooms
- three tsp flour
- Cream cheese, six ounces
- 1 1/2 cups non-dairy creamer, such as Mocha Mix
- 1/4 to 1/2 tsp of nutmeg
- Half a cup of freshly grated parmesan cheese
- 1 and a half zucchini, cut into little circles
- No-boil lasagna noodles, 1 box

Instructions

- Set oven temperature to 375 degrees.
- In a small pot, combine the chicken and stock; bring to a boil, then lower the heat and simmer until the chicken is cooked through and white. Chopped chicken will cook more quickly.
- In the meantime, add the onion, oregano, black pepper, and olive oil to a large sauté pan over medium heat. Sauté the onion for 5 minutes, or until it starts to soften.
- Pour wine into the pan, if using, and let it evaporate.

- Include mushrooms.
- To disperse the flavors, evenly sprinkle flour over the pan and stir. The pan's ingredients ought to appear clumpy.
- Give this a few minutes to fry (around three minutes).
- After breaking up the cream cheese, add it to the pan and stir again until it melts and is distributed evenly. (About two minutes)
- Stirring again, add the mocha mix to the pan slowly.
- The ingredients ought to be clump-free and thickening up. Continue stirring to break them up if they're still clumpy.
- Include the nutmeg.
- Add the parmesan cheese and simmer, stirring, for a further five minutes. The sauce should thicken as well.
- Remove chicken from pot (reserve the liquid) and using two forks, shred chicken apart, trying to keep pieces even.
- Put aside.
- To thin out the cream mixture, add in 1/2 cup of the reserved broth and stir occasionally for 2 minutes.
- Lay the lasagna sheets in the pan, cover with 1/3 of the sauce, then 1/2 of the chicken and 1/2 of the evenly distributed zucchini pieces; repeat layering, and finally drizzle with the remaining sauce.

- After 30 minutes of baking with the foil covered, take the foil off and bake for a few more minutes to achieve the required crispiness.

Nutritional Facts: Calories 453kcal, Carbohydrates 32g, Protein 23g, Sodium 277mg, Phosphorus 179mg, Potassium 317mg

110. LEMON TARRAGON CHICKEN

Cooking time: 25 mins   **Yield:** 8

Ingredients

- Two tsp margarine
- Eight medium chicken breast halves, skinless and boneless (about 0.5 pounds)
- Two cups of freshly cut mushrooms
- two minced cloves of garlic
- Three tsp of dry sherry
- ½ teaspoon of crushed dried tarragon
- Half a teaspoon of spice, lemon pepper
- 1 ½ cups chicken broth without sodium
- 1/4 cup of sour cream
- ⅓ cup of flour
- Noodles that have been heated up (not included in nutritional analysis)

Instructions

- In a 12-inch skillet set over medium heat, melt the margarine.
- Add chicken, mushrooms, garlic, sherry, tarragon, and lemon pepper spice.
- Cook, uncovered, stirring once, for 10 to 12 minutes, or until chicken is no longer pink.
- Using a slotted spoon, remove the chicken and mushrooms.
- Mix flour and chicken broth in a container with a tight-fitting cover, and shake to mix.
- Pour mixture into skillet. Cook over medium-high heat, stirring, until bubbling and thickened.
- Take approximately a quarter of the mixture out of the skillet and combine it with sour cream.
- Add the mixture back to the skillet with the chicken and mushrooms. Don't boil, just heat through.
- Place over freshly cooked noodles.

Nutritional Facts: Calories 237kcal, Fat 9g, Carbohydrates 8g, Protein 29g, Sodium 133mg, Calcium 28mg. Phosphorus 246mg, Potassium 419mg

111. SALISBURY STEAK

Cooking time: 23 mins   **Yield:** 6

Ingredients

- Two tablespoons of onion
- One clove of garlic
- Lean ground beef, 1 pound
- two white eggs
- Ten low-sodium soda crackers
- half a cup of low-sodium beef broth
- One tsp dried mustard
- One-half tablespoon of dehydrated parsley
- 1/4 tsp black pepper

Instructions

- Turn the oven on to 425°F.
- Dice onion and finely chop cloves of garlic. Break up crackers and weigh out half a cup.
- In a large bowl, mix all ingredients together.
- Create six hamburger patties out of the meat mixture.
- Cakes should be put in a baking dish.
- Bake for 20 minutes without cover.

Nutritional Facts: Calories 146kcal, Fat 6g, Carbohydrates 5g, Protein 18g, Sodium 104mg, Calcium 18mg. Phosphorus 160mg, Potassium 331mg

112. TURKEY WALDORF SALAD

Cooking time: 20 mins   **Yield:** 6

Ingredients

- Cooked 12-oz unsalted turkey breast
- three red apples, medium in size
- one cup of celery
- half a cup of onions
- 1/4 cup of mayonnaise
- Two tsp of apple juice

Instructions

- Cube up the turkey. Juice the apples and celery; finely slice the onion.
- Combine the turkey, apple, celery, and onion in a medium-sized bowl.
- Mix in apple juice and mayonnaise. Mix thoroughly by stirring.
- Until ready to serve, let cool.

Nutritional Facts: Calories 200kcal, Fat 11g, Carbohydrates 8g, Protein 17g, Sodium 128mg, Calcium 26mg. Phosphorus 136mg, Potassium 296mg

113.   CHICKEN WALDORF SALAD

Cooking time: 40 mins   **Yield:** 4

Ingredients

- Eight ounces of cooked and diced chicken or turkey
- half a cup of chopped apples
- half a cup of finely chopped celery
- two tsp of raisins

- Half a tablespoon of ground ginger, if desired
- Half a cup Miracle Whip

Instructions

- Blend until thoroughly combined.
- To mix the tastes, it is recommended to let it sit in the refrigerator for a bit.

Nutritional Facts: Calories 224kcal, Fat 15g, Carbohydrates 10g, Protein 14g, Sodium 233mg, Calcium 18mg. Phosphorus 129mg, Potassium 234mg

114.   CHICKEN WITH MUSHROOM SAUCE

Cooking time: 1hr 30mins   **Yield:** 8

Ingredients

- 1/4 cup of flour for all purposes
- Two tablespoons of mild sour cream
- 1 tablespoon mustard dijon
- 1 cup of chicken broth (choose a brand with no additional salt)
- 4 breasts of chicken, not "seasoned"
- 1/4 teaspoon of dried thyme
- One teaspoon of non-hydrogenated margarine
- 1 and a half cups chopped mushrooms
- three finely sliced green onions
- To taste, add freshly ground pepper and minced fresh parsley.

Instructions

- Stir together 2 tablespoons flour, mustard, sour cream, and 2 tablespoons chicken broth. Put aside.
- After seasoning the chicken with pepper and thyme, coat it with flour.
- In a large nonstick pan over medium-low heat, melt margarine.
- Cook chicken until no longer pink inside, about 5 minutes per side. Take out the chicken and keep it warm.
- Cook the mushrooms in the skillet for three minutes while stirring.
- Turn the heat up to high, add the remaining chicken broth, and boil for three minutes.
- Mix the sour cream mixture and stir in the green onions.
- After roughly three minutes, stir until thickened. Drizzle over the chicken, top with parsley and pepper, and serve.

Nutritional Facts: Calories 161kcal, Fat 4g, Carbohydrates 5g, Protein 25.4g, Sodium 99mg, Phosphorus 205mg, Potassium 289mg

115. GRILLED PINEAPPLE CHICKEN

Cooking time: 2hr 25mins   **Yield:** 4

Ingredients

- One cup of sherry, without sugar
- One cup of pineapple juice
- One spoonful of soy sauce with lower sodium
- Four pineapple rings
- one one-and-a-quarter-pound skinless, bone-in chicken breast

Instructions

- Put every ingredient—aside from the pineapple—into a zip-lock bag.
- Refrigerate and marinate overnight.
- After marinating, place the chicken on an indoor or outdoor grill and cook it for 15 to 20 minutes.
- Throw away any extra marinade.
- To reheat, place the pineapple on the grill for two minutes on each side during the final few minutes. Place atop every chicken breast.

Nutritional Facts: Calories 211kcal, Fat 3g, Carbohydrates 20g, Protein 26g, Sodium 215mg, Calcium 21mg. Phosphorus 198mg, Potassium 376mg

116. SPICY BEEF STIR-FRY

Cooking time: 35 mins   **Yield:** 4

Ingredients

- ¼ teaspoon sesame oil
- ½ teaspoon sugar,
- two teaspoons of separated cornstarch
- Two tablespoons of water, divided

- One large egg, beaten with three tablespoons of canola oil, 12 ounces of beef round tip separated, one green bell pepper, one cup of onions, and one ¼ teaspoon of ground red chili pepper (or to taste) sliced.
- One tablespoon of sherry
- Two teaspoons of low-sodium soy sauce
- Garnish optional: parsley

Instructions

- In a large bowl, combine 1 tablespoon cornstarch, 1 tablespoon water, 1 large egg, 1 tablespoon canola oil, and add the beef.   Give it a 20-minute marinade.
- Use another bowl to mix the remaining cornstarch and water. Put aside.
- The beef mixture is added to a skillet with the remaining two tablespoons of canola oil already heated. Cook until the meat starts to take on color.
- Add the onion, chili pepper, and green bell peppers. After adding the sherry, stir-fry everything for a minute. Stir in sugar, sesame oil, and soy sauce.
- Use a cornstarch and water mixture to thicken.
- Not required: Stir-fry beef with parsley as a garnish.

Nutritional Facts: Calories 261kcal, Fat 15g, Carbohydrates 10g, Protein 21g, Sodium 169mg, Calcium 26mg. Phosphorus 167mg, Potassium 313mg

117.   SOUTHWESTERN MEATLESS BURGER

Cooking time: 1hr 15mins   **Yield:** 6

Ingredients

- Six tsp olive oil
- one medium onion, chopped finely
- Half a cup of finely chopped red or green pepper
- half a cup of frozen or fresh corn
- two minced garlic cloves
- One medium-sized spaghetti squash makes approximately two cups of pureed squash, so use 1/2 cup.
- 1/4 cup extra-sharp cheddar cheese: the best flavor will come from a strong, high-quality cheese when ingested in tiny amounts.
- 1/4 cup nutritional yeast was used. This is an excellent product to have on hand since in some recipes it can take the place of the flavor of cheese. It can be purchased online or in the natural foods department of many supermarkets.
- half a cup of crushed low-sodium crackers or breadcrumbs
- half a cup of oatmeal
- Two tablespoons of freshly cut, finely parsley

- One dash of salt, according to taste
- 1 pinch to taste of freshly ground pepper
- 6–8 tortillas Although corn tortillas have the least amount of sodium, they must be thoroughly heated (frying, microwave, etc.)
- green salsa Make sure the green salsa you select is made using tomatillos or green chiles rather than green tomatoes by reading the ingredients on the label.
- Two cups of finely chopped lettuce
- Chopped fresh cilantro; optional sour cream

Instructions

- In a big nonstick skillet over medium heat, heat two teaspoons of oil. Add the onion and simmer for 5 to 7 minutes, stirring frequently, or until softened. Add the bell pepper, corn, garlic, chili powder, and cumin. Cook, stirring, for an additional two minutes or until fragrant. After moving to a big bowl, give it ten minutes or so to cool to room temperature.
- To the onion mixture, thoroughly combine the pureed spaghetti squash, cheese, oats, nutritional yeast, breadcrumbs, parsley, salt, and pepper. Using about 1/2 cup for each, shape the veggie mixture into six 1/2-inch-thick patties using wet palms.

- Turn the oven on to 325°F. Place flour or corn tortillas in a stack and cover with foil. Place in the oven to thoroughly heat, about 15 minutes. Alternately, place the tortillas between two damp paper towels and heat them in the microwave for 30 to 60 seconds on high, or until well heated.
- Cook 2 to 4 patties at a time in a large nonstick skillet over medium heat, adding 2 tablespoons of oil every batch, until browned and heated through, about 4 minutes per side. Adapt the heat as needed to ensure uniform browning. Although they don't have the same "crispy" shell that you might get with a pan-fry, we also had success baking them. Serve the patties right away, wrapped in tortillas and topped with salsa made with green chilies and tomatillos.
- Plan Ahead Advice: Get ready by completing Step 3. Patties can be frozen for up to three months or refrigerated for up to two days when individually wrapped. Refrigerate to thaw before using in cooking.
- The consistency of the mixture should resemble oatmeal cookie dough, which is a crucial component of this recipe. When flipped, the patties won't stay together if they are very moist and gooey. A small amount more oatmeal or bread crumbs can be added if your

mixture seems overly goopy or moist. You can also add an egg or some flavorless protein powder to a recipe if you're on dialysis and attempting to up your protein consumption.

Nutritional Facts: Calories 198kcal, Fat 8g, Carbohydrates 28g, Protein 6g, Sodium 121mg, Calcium 88mg, Potassium 253mg

118.   SOFT TACOS WITH MEXICAN SEASONING

Cooking time: 35 mins   **Yield:** 7

Ingredients

- One recipe (included in the Sauces & Stew section) for Mexican Seasoning
- Five tablespoons of onion
- two cups of lettuce
- One pound of ground beef
- 1/2 cup tomato sauce reduced in sodium
- Fourteen six-inch flour tortillas
- Shredded five tablespoons of strong cheddar cheese
- Five spoonfuls of sour cream

Instructions

- Prepare the recipe for Mexican Seasoning.
- Chop the lettuce and onion.
- Grind the ground meat and drain. Stir in the low-sodium tomato sauce and

the seasoning combination. Turn the heat to medium. Reheat the tortillas.

- To put together soft tacos, take one flour tortilla, top it with 1/4 cup of ground beef that has been seasoned, 1 teaspoon each of cheese, onion, and sour cream, and top it with lettuce, if preferred.

Nutritional Facts: Calories 340kcal, Fat 15g, Carbohydrates 32g, Protein 19g, Sodium 494mg, Calcium 143mg. Phosphorus 276mg, Potassium 422mg

119.   UPPER PENINSULA PASTIES

Cooking time: 1hr 35mins   **Yield:** 8

Ingredients

- 1/4 cup of carrot
- one-fourth cup onion
- One pound of ground steak
- one-fourth cup of frozen corn
- One-fourth cup of frozen peas
- One tablespoon of sodium-reduced Sauce from Worcestershire
- One tsp black pepper
- A single tsp of dried thyme
- 15-oz box with two crusts Refrigerated, rolled, and unbaked pie crust
- One white egg
- Eight tsp of ketchup

Instructions

- Set oven temperature to 375°F. Follow the instructions on the package and let the pie crust stand at room temperature.
- Chop onion and dice carrot.
- Over medium heat, brown ground sirloin in a large skillet. After draining, set away.
- Put a carrot on a plate for the microwave. Cover, add 1 tablespoon of water, and simmer for 2 minutes on high. Microwave for two minutes after adding the frozen corn and peas. Empty.
- In a bowl, mix the meat, veggies, onion, Worcestershire sauce, black pepper, and thyme to make the filling.
- Pie crusts should be unrolled on a lightly floured surface. Each pie crust should have four parts.
- Place a quarter cup of the filling on half of each pie crust half. Use a tiny bit of milk or egg white to lightly moisten the edges of the pie crust.
- Over the filling, fold the remaining pie shell. Using a fork, pinch edges to seal. Score the tops of the pastries with slits. Apply a final coat of egg white on top. Place on a large, ungreased baking sheet.
- Bake until the crust is golden brown, 15 to 20 minutes. Cool on wire racks a little.

- Put a tsp of ketchup on each pasty.

Nutritional Facts: Calories 354kcal, Fat 22g, Carbohydrates 28g, Protein 11g, Sodium 382mg, Calcium 12mg. Phosphorus 72mg, Potassium 214mg

120.   SWEDISH MEATBALLS

Cooking time: 50 mins   **Yield:** 24

Ingredients

- half a cup of onions
- Two big eggs
- Three pounds of ground beef
- One tablespoon of canola oil
- One cup raw oatmeal
- 1/2 cup beef broth with low sodium
- 1 tablespoon dried dill
- Twice as much dried thyme
- One-fourth teaspoon of nutmeg
- One-fourth teaspoon ground allspice
- 1/4 tsp black pepper
- Three tsp unsalted butter
- Three tablespoons of all-purpose white flour
- Two cups beef broth with reduced sodium
- one-third cup water

Instructions

- Warm the oven up to 375°F.
- Finely chop the onion. Beat the eggs.

- In a large bowl, combine the first 11 ingredients; stir well to combine.
- Place on a baking sheet and roll into 1-inch balls.
- Bake meatballs for 10 to 15 minutes, or until done.
- To create sauce, heat butter in a big saucepan.
- Add the flour, water, broth with reduced sodium, and the last tablespoon of dried thyme. Cook over medium heat, stirring until thickened.
- Put the meatballs in the sauce and reduce the heat to maintain their warmth, or you can use a slow cooker on low heat or a covered warming dish.

Nutritional Facts: Calories 172kcal, Fat 11g, Carbohydrates 4g, Protein 11g, Sodium 93mg, Calcium 19mg. Phosphorus 91mg, Potassium 140mg

121. BAKED PORK CHOPS

Cooking time: 23 mins   **Yield:** 6

Ingredients

- Half a cup of all-purpose flour
- One big egg
- one-fourth cup water
- Three quarters a cup of cornflakes
- 6 center cut pork chops, 3-1/2 ounces each
- Half a tablespoon of unsalted butter
- One tsp of paprika
- 1/4 tsp salt
- Six peach halves in juice cans

Instructions

- Preheat the oven to 350 °F.
- In a plate or flat shallow pan, combine flour.
- In a shallow bowl, beat together the egg and water mixture. On a small plate, spread out the cornflake crumbs.
- Coat the pork chops with flour dredging. After dipping each chop into the egg mixture, coat it with cornflake crumbs.
- Lay chops on a baking sheet coated with cooking spray that doesn't stick. Pour over some melted margarine.
- Sprinkle chops with salt and paprika, then chill for a minimum of one hour.
- Bake pork chops until done, about 40 minutes.
- Before serving, place a drained peach half on top of each pork chop that has been grilled on a grill pan.

Nutritional Facts: Calories 282kcal, Fat 10g, Carbohydrates 25g, Protein 23g, Sodium 263mg, Calcium 28mg. Phosphorus 203mg, Potassium 394mg

122. EASY BEEF BURGERS

Cooking time: 20 mins   **Yield:** 4

Ingredients

- 450g (18 oz) of lean minced be
- 1 small (60g / 2 ½ oz) dried mixed herb
- ½ teaspoon black pepper
- ¼ teaspoon beaten egg; 1 medium

Instructions

- Combine the beaten egg, chopped meat, onion, mixed herbs, and black pepper.
- Split the ingredients into four equal parts, then form each into a round, flat cake.
- Grill for approximately ten minutes on each side, occasionally pressing to release any juice.

Nutritional Facts: Calories 238kcal, Fat 16g, Carbohydrates 0.5g, Protein 23g, Sodium 200mg, Phosphorus 187mg, Potassium 274mg

123. HAWAIIAN-STYLE SLOW-COOKED PULLED PORK

Cooking time: 4hrs 10mins   **Yield:** 16

Ingredients

- 4 lbs. of roast pork
- ½ teaspoon of black pepper, ground
- one-half teaspoon paprika
- One tsp powdered onion
- One-half teaspoon of powdered garlic

- two tsp liquid smoke
- Garnish optional: (Radish or pickled red onions) One red onion or four radishes, one-quarter cup white vinegar, and one-tsp sugar

Instructions

- In a small bowl, mix together garlic powder, onion powder, paprika, and black pepper.
- Apply the spice mixture to the pork's whole surface. Put the pork in a crock-pot or slow cooker. Add a dash of liquid smoke.
- Fill the slow cooker or crock-pot with enough water to reach a depth of ¼ to ½". Simmer for 4-5 hours on high.
- Take the pork out of the cooking liquid and use two forks to shred the meat.

Nutritional Facts: Calories 285kcal, Fat 21g, Carbohydrates 1g, Protein 20g, Sodium 54mg, Calcium 9mg. Phosphorus 230mg, Potassium 380mg

124. MEDITERRANEAN LAMB PATTIES

Cooking time: 30 mins   **Yield:** 4

Ingredients

- One pound of lamb, ground
- One whole egg
- 1/4 cup of breadcrumbs, panko

- 1/4 cup finely chopped onions
- One garlic clove, cut finely
- One teaspoon of dried mint (or dried oregano)
- half a teaspoon of pepper, ground
- Half a cup of crumbled feta cheese

Instructions

- Mix all the ingredients together thoroughly in a sizable bowl.
- Make four equal-sized patties that are roughly 1/2 inch thick.
- Heat a sizable nonstick skillet to medium-high temperature.
- Once the patties are browned, add them and continue cooking on high for 5 minutes on each side before lowering the heat.
- Make sure the patties are fully cooked when the internal temperature reaches 160 degrees or when they are no longer pink in the center.

Nutritional Facts: Calories 305kcal, Carbohydrates 5g, Protein 19g, Sodium 229mg, Phosphorus 74mg, Potassium 45mg

125. BOURBON-GLAZED SKIRT STEAK

Cooking time: 1hr 30mins   **Yield:** 8

Ingredients

Bourbon Glaze

- Diced shallots, ¼ cup
- Three tablespoons of cold, diced unsalted butter
- 1/2 cup dark brown sugar
- 1 cup bourbon
- Two tsp Dijon mustard
- 1 tsp ground pepper

Skirt steak

- Grape seed oil, two tablespoons
- Half a teaspoon of dried oregano
- one-half teaspoon of paprika
- One tsp black pepper
- One tablespoon of vinegar made from red wine
- Two pounds of skirt steak

Instructions

Whiskey Glaze

- Shallots should be browned in 1 tablespoon of butter in a small pot over medium-high heat.
- Turn down the heat to low, take the pan off the burner, pour in the bourbon, and put it back on.
- Cook until reduced by about one third, 10 to 15 minutes.
- Stir in mustard, black pepper, and brown sugar until bubbling.
- After turning off the heat, thoroughly mix in the remaining 2 tablespoons of cold, cubed butter, stirring all the while.

Skirt Steak

- Combine the first five ingredients in a gallon-sized resealable bag, then add steaks and give it a good shake.
- Give the steaks 30 to 45 minutes to marinate in the bag at room temperature.
- Take the steaks out of the bag, grill them for 15 to 20 minutes on each side, then take them out and let them rest for ten minutes to rest.
- Cut in half and serve with a drizzle of sauce, or leave whole, coat with glaze, and broil for four to six minutes, or until desired texture is achieved.

Nutritional Facts: Calories 409kcal, Fat 22g, Carbohydrates 8g, Protein 24g, Sodium 152mg, Calcium 22mg. Phosphorus 171mg, Potassium 283mg

126.   CHILI CON CARNE

Cooking time: 1br 10mins   **Yield:** 8

Ingredients

- half a cup of onions
- one celery stalk
- Half a cup of green bell pepper
- Thin ground beef, 1 and a half pounds
- 16 ounces of low-sodium stewed tomatoes
- One tablespoon of canola oil
- two tsp of chili powder

- 1/2 cup of water

Instructions

- Chop the bell pepper, celery, and onion.
- Warm up a big skillet over medium heat. Add the oil, bell pepper, onion, and celery and cook until soft but not browned.
- Cook the ground beef until it turns brown, breaking it up into small pieces.
- Blend tomatoes in a blender and add to the beef. Stir in the water and chili powder. Mix well; turn down the heat.
- Simmer for a few hours.

Nutritional Facts: Calories 190kcal, Fat 10g, Carbohydrates 5g, Protein 20g, Sodium 116mg, Calcium 38mg. Phosphorus 180mg, Potassium 450mg

127.   PORK PASTIES

Cooking time: 60 mins   **Yield:** 6

Ingredients

Regarding the Pastry

- Two cups of all-purpose flour
- 1/2 cup whole wheat flour
- 1/2 teaspoon salt
- 1 cup unsalted butter, cooled and cubed
- half a cup of cold water

Regarding the Filling

- One pound of finely chopped lean pork
- One cup of peeled and coarsely chopped carrots
- One cup of peeled and finely chopped potatoes
- half a cup of peas
- 1/2 cup chicken broth with minimal sodium and 1 tbsp olive oil
- One little onion, diced finely
- two minced garlic cloves
- A single tsp of dried thyme
- To taste, add salt and pepper.

Instructions

- Mix the whole wheat flour, all-purpose flour, and salt together in a big bowl.
- Using a pastry cutter or your fingers, add the chilled, chopped butter and stir until the mixture resembles coarse crumbs.
- Add the cold water little by little and stir until the dough comes together. Press it into a disk, wrap it in plastic wrap, and place it in the fridge for at least half an hour.
- Turn the oven on to 375°F, or 190°C.
- Heat the olive oil in a pan over medium heat.
- Add the minced garlic and onions, and cook until they become tender.
- Cook the chopped pork until it turns brown. Add the potatoes, carrots, green peas, and dried thyme and stir.
- Once the vegetables are soft, add the low-sodium chicken broth and boil. To taste, add salt and pepper for seasoning.
- On a surface dusted with flour, roll out the chilled pastry to a thickness of about 1/8 inch. Cut out circles with a diameter of around 6-7 inches.
- Leaving a small border around the borders, spoon a substantial dollop of the pork and vegetable mixture onto one half of each pastry circle. Using the pastry, fold it over the filling to form a semicircle. Using a fork, crimp the edges after pressing them to seal.
- Transfer the pasties to a parchment paper-lined baking sheet. Bake for about 25 to 30 minutes, or until the pastry is golden brown, in a preheated oven.
- Before serving, let the pasties cool somewhat. Savor these tasty and filling kidney-friendly pork pasties for dinner.

Nutritional Facts: Calories 400kcal, Fat 20g, Carbohydrates 40g, Protein 15g, Sodium: varies, Calcium 40mg, Phosphorus 200mg, Potassium 400mg

128.   TACOS

Cooking time: 30 mins   **Yield:** 6

Ingredients

- Six corn tortilla shells
- Lean ground beef, half a pound
- ,\One tablespoon of canola oil
- One cup of chopped onion, split for usage
- one minced clove of garlic
- One tsp of chili powder
- half a teaspoon of pepper, black
- 1/4 tsp ground cumin
- One-fourth teaspoon Tabasco® sauce
- one-third cup of shredded lettuce
- Six tablespoons of chopped tomato
- Six tablespoons of shredded sharp cheddar cheese

Instructions

- Over medium heat, cook the ground beef in a large frying skillet. Thoroughly drain, take out of the pan, and reserve.
- Warm up the pan's oil. Cook until transparent after adding 1/2 cup minced onion. Stir and sauté the garlic for one minute.
- Return the cooked beef to the pan. Add the Tabasco® sauce, pepper, cumin, and chili powder and stir. Take off the heat and get your tacos ready.
- Put a quarter cup of the meat mixture into each taco shell. Add two teaspoons of lettuce, one tablespoon of each of the leftover onion, tomato, and cheese on top.

Nutritional Facts: Calories 240kcal, Fat 16g, Carbohydrates 14g, Protein 10g, Sodium 182mg, Calcium 85mg. Phosphorus 135mg, Potassium 214mg

129.   BROCCOLI AND BEEF STIR-FRY

Cooking time: 30 mins   **Yield:** 4

Ingredients

- two cloves of garlic
- One Roma tomato, medium
- Eight ounces of raw, lean sirloin meat
- One dozen frozen broccoli ounces stir-fried mix of vegetables
- two tsp of peanut oil
- 1/4 cup chicken broth with minimal sodium
- One tablespoon of cornflour
- Two teaspoons of soy sauce with lower sodium
- Two cups of cooked white or brown rice

Instructions

- Dice the Roma tomato and garlic cloves. Slice the beef thinly.

- Thaw frozen stir-fry veggie blend in the microwave for three to four minutes on the defrost setting.
- Heat the oil in a fry pan or wok and sauté the garlic until it becomes aromatic. Add vegetable blend and stir-fry for 5 minutes or until cooked through. Take out of the pan and place aside.
- Add the beef to the same pan. Cook for about 7 minutes, or until beef is cooked to your liking.
- In a bowl, mix soy sauce, cornstarch, and chicken broth to make the sauce.
- Include the tomato, sauce, and cooked veggies in the skillet with the beef. The sauce should thicken with heat and stirring.
- Serve the dish over half a cup of rice.

Nutritional Facts: Calories 373kcal, Fat 17g, Carbohydrates 37g, Protein 18g, Sodium 351mg, Calcium 62mg. Phosphorus 255mg, Potassium 555mg

130. ONION STEAK

Cooking time: 1hr 50mins   **Yield:** 8

Ingredients

- One and a half pounds of ½-inch-thick round steak
- One-fourth cup flour
- one-eighth teaspoon of pepper
- two teaspoons olive oil
- one cup of water
- 1 tablespoon vinegar
- one minced garlic clove
- One bay leaf, ¼ teaspoon of crushed dried thyme
- three medium-sized onions, sliced

Instructions

- Divide the steak into 8 equal halves.
- Mix pepper and flour together, then pound into the meat.
- Heat oil in a skillet on medium high heat. Meat should be browned on both sides. Take out of the skillet and place aside.
- In the skillet, mix the water, vinegar, garlic, bay leaf, and thyme. Heat till boiling.
- Add the meat to this mixture, then top with the onion slices.
- Simmer for one hour with a lid on.

Nutritional Facts: Calories 184kcal, Fat 7g, Carbohydrates 4g, Protein 26g, Sodium 57mg, Calcium 19mg. Phosphorus 236mg, Potassium 342mg

CHAPTER 8

SEAFOOD & FISH OPTIONS

131.   FISH TACOS

Cooking time: 55 mins   **Yield:** 6

Ingredients

- 1-1/2 cups of cabbage
- Half a cup red onion, half a handful of cilantro
- One clove of garlic
- two limes
- One-pound filets of cod
- half a teaspoon of cumin powder
- Half a teaspoon of red pepper flakes
- 1/4 tsp black pepper
- One tablespoon of olive oil
- one-half cup mayonnaise
- One-fourth cup sour cream
- two tsp milk
- 12 six-inch corn tortillas

Instructions

- Chop the cilantro, onion, and cabbage, and shred it. Put aside. Dice the garlic.
- Squeeze the juice of 1/2 a lime over the fish filets that have been placed on a platter. Add olive oil, chili powder, cumin, black pepper, and minced garlic to the filets. After turning the filets to coat them with marinade, chill them for a half hour or more.

- Combine mayonnaise, sour cream, milk, and half a lime juice to make salsa blanca. After giving everything a quick stir, chill in the refrigerator.
- Preheat the oven to broil. Use foil to cover the broiler pan. Fish should be broiled for about ten minutes, or until the flesh turns opaque and white and the fish flakes readily. Take the fish out of the oven, let it cool down a bit, and then break it into big pieces.
- One by one, reheat the corn tortillas in a pan until they are tender and warm. To keep them warm, cover them with a fresh dish towel.
- Place a slice of fish on a tortilla, then top with cabbage, red onion, cilantro, and lime wedges to make the tacos. If you want, add hot sauce.

132.   HONEY SPICE RUBBED SALMON HONEY SPICE RUBBED SALMON

Cooking time: 22 mins   **Yield:** 4

Ingredients

- three tsp honey
- three-quarter teaspoons of lemon peel
- half a teaspoon of pepper, black

- half a teaspoon of powdered garlic
- One tsp warm water
- 16-ounce filets of salmon
- Two tsp olive oil
- three cups of arugula

Instructions

- In a small bowl, combine honey, grated lemon peel, crushed pepper, garlic powder, and boiling water; whisk to combine. Rub mixture over salmon filets with gloved hands.
- In a skillet over medium heat, warm the olive oil. Salmon filets with spice rub should be added and cooked for 4 minutes. Using a spatula, flip the filets slowly.
- Lower the heat to medium-low and continue cooking for another 4 to 6 minutes, or until the fish flakes easily with a fork and becomes opaque throughout.
- Place half a cup of arugula onto every plate. Top arugula with a salmon filet and serve.

133.   FISH PAPILLOTE

Cooking time: 40 mins   **Yield:** 4

Ingredients

- 4 fish pieces, each weighing about 120 g

- two carrots
- One stalk celery
- pepper
- One lemon
- Four parchment paper sheets

Instructions

- Put a salmon slice on a piece of parchment paper.
- Wash and peel the carrots. For five minutes, cook the carrots in a lot of water.
- Add a couple carrot sticks and celery to each papillote.
- Add some pepper and a lemon slice. Put the papillote away.
- Bake or use a steamer for 15 minutes of cooking.

134.   LOUISIANA SHRIMP AND CRAB GUMBO

Cooking time: 1hr 30mins   **Yield:** 6

Ingredients

- One medium green bell pepper
- One medium onion
- One clove of garlic
- One leafy celery stalk
- Four green onion tops
- 1/4 cup canola oil
- 1/4 cup fresh parsley
- Six tablespoons of flour (all-purpose)

- three cups of water
- Four cups chicken broth reduced in sodium
- 8 ounces of raw shrimp
- Six ounces of crab meat
- 1/4 tsp black pepper
- 1 tspn of hot Tabasco® sauce
- three cups of boiled rice

Instructions

- Cut the bell pepper, onion, celery, garlic, green onion tops, and parsley into pieces.
- Heat the oil and flour in a big skillet over medium heat to produce a roux. Until the flour has a pecan color, stir continuously.
- To the roux, add the bell pepper, onion, garlic, celery, and one cup of water. Vegetables should be covered and cooked over very low heat until soft.
- Turn the heat up to high and stir in 4 cups low-sodium chicken broth and 2 cups water. Simmer for five minutes.
- Add the shrimp and crab meat after lowering the heat to medium. Simmer for ten minutes.
- Add parsley and tops of green onions. For five minutes, simmer over low heat.
- Serve over rice and season with pepper and spicy sauce.

135.   FIESTA TILAPIA CEVICHE

Cooking time: 38 mins   **Yield:** 8

Ingredients

- 1.5 pounds of fresh filets of tilapia
- One cup of red onions
- Half a cup of red bell pepper
- one-fourth cup cilantro
- One cup of pineapple
- Two tsp of canola oil
- 1/4 tsp black pepper
- One-and-a-quarter cups of liquid lime.
- 48 unsalted toppings on saltine crackers

Instructions

- Chop the cilantro, bell pepper, and onion. Cut the pineapple into dice. Cut tilapia into little pieces.
- For 3 minutes on each side, broil the tilapia cubes under high heat.
- After letting the tilapia cool for five minutes, carefully combine it with fresh lime juice. Ensure that every tilapia piece is fully submerged in the lime juice.
- Add the cooked tilapia to a mixture that includes bell pepper, onion, cilantro, pineapple, black pepper, and canola oil.
- To let the food marinade for at least two hours, cover and refrigerate.

- Accompany each serving with six unsalted saltine crackers.

136. SHRIMP, SUGAR SNAP PEA SALAD AND WASABI-LIME VINAIGRETTE

Cooking time: 40mins **Yield:** 6

Ingredients

- One pound of big, peeled shrimp
- Two cups of clipped snap peas
- One cup of drained water chestnuts
- One cup of sprouting beans
- Wasabi-Lime Dressing
- one-half cup of vegetable oil
- 1/4 cup vinegar made from rice wine
- One tablespoon of lime juice
- three teaspoons of wasabi powder
- One teaspoon of sugar
- 1 tsp finely chopped ginger
- 1/2 teaspoon minced garlic

Instructions

- Heat up a big saucepan of water until it boils.
- Add the shrimp and snap peas, and simmer for about 2 minutes, or until the shrimp become pink.
- To prevent overcooking, quickly move the shrimp and snap peas to cooled water and drain.

- Whisk together all the ingredients to make the vinaigrette.
- Serve the vinaigrette-tossed shrimp, snap peas, water chestnuts, and bean sprouts.
- Because wasabi powder is really spicy, it's best to use less of it!

137. CRUNCHY OVEN-FRIED CATFISH

Cooking time: 35 mins **Yield:** 4

Ingredients

- One white egg
- Half a cup of all-purpose flour
- one-fourth cup cornmeal
- 1/4 cup of breadcrumbs, panko
- One teaspoon of salt-free Seasoning from Cajun
- One-pound filets of catfish

Instructions

- Preheat the oven to 450°F.
- Apply cooking spray to the flat, nonstick baking sheet's surface.
- In a small dish, beat the egg white until very soft peaks form. Don't beat yourself up.
- On a piece of wax paper, spread flour.
- Add the panko, Cajun seasoning, and cornmeal to a different wax paper sheet.

- Cut the catfish filet into four equal pieces. Shake off any extra flour after dipping the fish in it.
- Fish coated with flour is dipped in egg white and then rolled in the cornmeal mixture.
- Put the fish on the baking pan and proceed with steps 6 through 9 for each filet of fish.
- Apply cooking spray to the tops of the fish filets and bake for 10 to 12 minutes, or until the fish is sizzling and the bottoms of the filets are browned. After taking the pan out of the oven, flip the fish over.
- Put the fish back in the oven and bake it for a further five minutes or so, or until the filets are crisp and golden.

138. ROASTED SALMON FILETS

Cooking time: 20 mins **Yield:** 2

Ingredients

- 10 ounces of salmon (two skin-on filets)
- 1/4 tsp of freshly cracked black pepper
- One tablespoon of olive oil
- One lemon (zest and juice)
- Four fresh cilantro sprigs

Instructions

- Place the salmon filets on the aluminum foil-covered toaster oven tray.
- Rub fish with olive oil, fresh lemon juice, zest, and black pepper.
- Add freshly chopped cilantro on top.
- Toasted salmon should be cooked on a dark roast (full circle) for 6 and a half minutes.
- Take out the toaster oven tray, squeeze some lemon over the salmon, and serve.

139. SALMON STEAKS WITH HERB DRESSING

Cooking time: 30 mins **Yield:** 6

Ingredients

- three-quarter cup of mayonnaise
- Three tsp of buttermilk
- Three tablespoons of raw dill
- One tablespoon of newly chopped chives
- two lemons
- Ten whole black peppercorns and one medium onion
- three parsley sprigs
- two bay leaves
- Half a teaspoon of salt
- Two pounds of salmon steaks

Instructions

- Halve a lemon into six slices and reserve. Zest half a teaspoon from the other lemon's peel. Juice five teaspoons of lemon. Chop the parsley and dill weed, and slice the onion.
- To make the dressing, put the mayonnaise or salad dressing, buttermilk, chives, 2 tablespoons dill weed, lemon zest, and 1 tablespoon lemon juice in a small mixing bowl. Once covered, let it sit for at least an hour.
- Combine the onion, peppercorns, parsley, bay leaves, salt, and the remaining 4 tablespoons of lemon juice with 1-1/2 cups of water in a 12-inch skillet. When boiling, add the fish steaks. When testing the fish with a fork, cook it for 8 to 12 minutes (or 12 to 18 minutes if it's frozen).
- Top salmon steaks with dressing and serve. Add the remaining dill weed and lemon wedges as garnish.

140. MEDITERRANEAN STYLE MUSSELS

Cooking time: 35 mins   **Yield:** 4

Ingredients

- Two tablespoons of unsalted butter
- one small (70 grams) of thinly sliced onions
- two cloves of minced garlic
- two cups of white wine (white Burgundy was used for the nutrient calculations).
- 12 ounces of uncooked, cleaned, and debearded mussels
- a quarter cup of chopped parsley

Instructions

- In a big, deep skillet set over medium-low heat, melt butter.
- Add the garlic and onion, and cook for five minutes.
- Put the mussels, wine, and parsley in and increase the heat to medium for two minutes, or until the wine starts to bubble.
- Put a lid on it and reduce the heat so that it simmers. Sauté the mussels until they open.
- In a big bowl, serve mussels in their shells. Cover the mussels with the sauce.

141. BAKED FISH

Cooking time: 35 mins   **Yield:** 4

Ingredients

- One-pound filets of cod
- Two tsp olive oil
- half a teaspoon of cumin powder
- half a teaspoon of rosemary, ground
- half a teaspoon of pepper, black

Instructions

- Set oven temperature to 350°F.
- Fish filets should be flattened and turned several times in olive oil to ensure full coating.
- Season fish with seasonings.
- Put inside of a baking dish.
- Bake for 20 to 25 minutes, or until a fork can easily pierce the fish.

142.   CRAB CAKES

Cooking time: 40 mins   **Yield:** 6

Ingredients

- one-third cup bell pepper
- one-fourth cup onion
- Six Ritz® salt-free crackers
- One big egg
- One pound of crab meat
- a quarter cup of low-fat mayonnaise
- One tablespoon of mustard powder
- One tsp black pepper
- One tablespoon of recently harvested parsley
- two tsp lemon juice
- One spoonful of powdered garlic
- a little pinch of cayenne
- Three teaspoons of olive oil

Instructions

- Chop the onion and bell pepper finely. Break apart the crackers.

- Mix all of the aforementioned ingredients, excluding the oil, and form into six patties.
- In a skillet over medium heat, heat the oil.
- Burgers should be cooked for around 4 to 5 minutes, or until browned.
- After about 4 minutes, flip the patties over and cook the other side until browned.
- Warm up and serve.

143.   CEVICHE CARIBE

Cooking time: 1hr 50mins   **Yield:** 6

Ingredients

- 12 large frozen, cooked, and peeled shrimp
- Two onions green
- One medium-sized tomato
- One medium-sized yellow banana pepper
- One tiny, recently-picked fiery chili pepper
- two tsp of raw cilantro
- three tsp lime juice
- A couple of tablespoons of pure white vinegar
- one tsp powdered garlic
- One cup of raw pineapple
- One tablespoon of olive oil

Instructions

- After thawing, remove the shrimp's tails. Dice into little pieces.
- Add the green onions, tomato, peppers, and cilantro to a food processor. Pulse on and off to chop the ingredients to a very coarse consistency. The texture should be chunky. Stir in the vinegar, garlic powder, and lime juice.
- Transfer the mixture to a serving bowl and stir in the olive oil and chopped shrimp.
- Take the fresh pineapple and core it. Pulse to chop to a coarse consistency after placing in the food processor. Toss the pineapple into the bowl with the veggies and shrimp. Combine ingredients by folding them together.
- Let it cool for at least half an hour before serving.

144.   LEMON DILL FISH

Cooking time: 30 mins   **Yield:** 4

Ingredients

- Twelve ounces (360 grams) Fish filet
- 1 tablespoon (15 mL) of lemon juice
- 3 tablespoons (50 mL) of fresh dill
- 1 tablespoon (15 mL) of melted margarine

Instructions

- Combine margarine, lemon juice, and dill.

- Apply a coat on the filet.
- Transfer the fish to a 9-inch (2.5-liter) pan and cover with the leftover sauce.
- Fish should flake easily with a fork and no longer be transparent after baking at 325°F (160°C).

145.   TUNA FISHCAKES

Cooking time: 1hr 30mins   **Yield:** 4

Ingredients

- One medium-sized baked potato, cooked to a cup
- three 6-oz tuna cans, rinsed and drained
- One whole egg
- 1/4 cup of breadcrumbs, panko
- 1/4 cup finely chopped onions
- 2 teaspoons of seasoning without salt
- half a teaspoon of pepper, ground
- One-fourth teaspoon cayenne (optional)
- One spoonful of mustard dijon
- Two tsp finely chopped capers
- One tablespoon of vegetable oil for the lemon wedge garnish

Instructions

- After giving the potato a fork poke, microwave it on high for five minutes, or until it is tender.

- Once cooked, remove the insides and use a fork to mash. Toss the potato skin.
- Mix all the ingredients together in a big bowl.
- Make 4 equal-sized patties that are roughly 0.5 inches thick.
- Heat the oil in a big skillet over medium-high heat.
- Add patties and cook on low for about 5 minutes on each side, or until browned.

CHAPTER 9

VEGETABLES & SALAD RECIPES

146. BASIL OIL

Cooking time: 15 mins   **Yield:** 16

Ingredients

- One and a half cups of fresh basil
- One cup of vegetable or olive oil

Instructions

- One and a half cups of finely packed fresh basil leaves should be rinsed and drained.
- Using a cloth, pat dry the leaves.
- Add 1 cup of olive or vegetable oil and the basil leaves to a blender or food processor. Process just until leaves are chopped finely; do not purée.
- Over medium heat, pour mixture into a 1- to 1-1/2-quart pan. For 3–4 minutes, or until the oil bubbles around the pan's edges and reaches 165 degrees on a thermometer, stir from time to time. To ensure that all germs in the combination are killed, make sure the oil is heated to this level.
- Take off the heat and allow it to cool for approximately one hour.
- Place two layers of cheesecloth over a fine wire strainer and place it over a small dish.
- Fill the strainer with the oil mixture.

- Once the oil has passed through, massage the basil gently into the leftover oil.
- Throw out the basil.
- Oil can be served or kept for up to three months in the refrigerator in an airtight container. When refrigerated, the olive oil may harden slightly, but it will liquefy fast when returning to room temperature.

147. HERB PESTO

Cooking time: 10 mins   **Yield:** 1½ cups

Ingredients

- One cup of tightly packed, fresh basil leaves
- Half a cup of freshly packed oregano and parsley leaves, respectively
- two cloves of garlic
- one-fourth cup olive oil
- two tsp freshly extracted lemon juice

Instructions

- In a food processor, pulse the garlic, parsley, oregano, and basil for about 3 minutes, or until very finely chopped.

- Until a thick paste develops, drizzle the olive oil into the pesto, scraping along the sides at least once.
- After adding the lemon juice, pulse to fully blend.
- For up to a week, keep the pesto refrigerated in a covered container.

148.   IRISH COLCANNON

Cooking time: 60 mins   **Yield:** 6

Ingredients

- Three medium parsnips (288g), sliced
- one medium russet potato (85g), quartered
- three tablespoons of divided olive oil
- one cup of kale
- one cup of shredded green cabbage
- one medium sized onion, diced
- two cloves of garlic, minced
- one and a half cups (240g) of frozen green peas
- freshly ground black pepper to taste
- (Optional) sea salt

Instructions

- Put the potato and cut parsnips in a big pot of water and heat it until it boils. Simmer over high heat for 15 minutes or until the food is soft.
- Using a strainer, remove the cooked vegetables. Keep the leftover cooking liquid in the pot aside.
- Mash the veggies with 2 tablespoons olive oil and 1/3 cup cooking liquid in a small basin. To get rid of lumps, add as much extra cooking liquid as necessary. A hand blender is an additional option.
- Store the mixture of mashed parsnips on a foil-covered platter.
- Toss in the chopped kale and shredded cabbage with the parsnip water. Cook until cabbage is slightly wilted, a few minutes.
- After completely draining, add the greens and cabbage back to the pot. Put a lid on it and set aside.
- A big skillet filled with one tablespoon of olive oil is heated over medium heat. Cook the minced garlic and onion until they become tender.
- When the cabbage and greens are in the saucepan, add the sautéed onions and garlic. Put the peas in.
- Arrange the potato and parsnip mash in the middle of a shallow dish or serving bowl. Add the cooked vegetables and stir. If used, season with salt and pepper.
- Warm it up as a side dish or have it for lunch with some crusty bread and green salad.

149. SWEET KOREAN LENTILS

Cooking time: 15 mins   **Yield:** 4

Ingredients

- Sauce
- two cups of water
- one-fourth cup of coconut aminos
- Two tablespoons of brown sugar
- two chopped garlic cloves
- 1 inch of finely chopped fresh ginger
- Crushed red pepper, use 1/4 to 1/2 teaspoon. If you like a little heat, use 1/2 teaspoon.
- One tsp of sesame oil
- Lentils
- One tablespoon of olive oil
- cut half of a yellow onion
- One cup red lentils and two chopped green onions

Instructions

- Combine all sauce ingredients in a large measuring cup or jar.
- In a medium-sized or larger pot, heat the oil over medium-high heat. When the onion is soft and starting to brown, add it and sauté it for three to five minutes.
- After adding the lentils and sauce, slowly bring it to a boil. For 8 to 10 minutes, cook while covered and reduced to a simmer. Most of the liquid will have been absorbed by the delicate lentils.
- Divide the lentils into four halves and top with green onions.

150. STUFFED POBLANO PEPPER

Cooking time: 1hr 10mins   Yield: 8

Ingredients

- Two 15-ounce low-sodium pinto bean cans, rinsed and drained
- 1 cup water
- a single tablespoon of canola oil
- one sliced onion
- four minced garlic cloves
- One tablespoon of ground cumin
- One teaspoon of dried oregano
- One teaspoon of chili powder
- two limes, juiced and zest
- 1/8 tsp cayenne pepper (or more if you enjoy spicy food!)
- 1/4 tsp salt
- two cups of corn, frozen
- One cup of shredded Monterey Jack cheese
- One cup of shredded cheddar cheese
- minced half a cup of fresh cilantro
- Eight poblano peppers
- One cup of quartered cherry tomatoes
- One tablespoon of olive oil

Instructions

- In a bowl, mix one can of beans with some water. Mash until mainly smooth. Put aside.
- In a 12-inch skillet, preheat canola oil over medium-high heat. Add the onion and simmer for about 5 minutes, or until tender. Add the lime zest, chili powder, garlic, cumin, oregano, salt, and cayenne. Cook for about 30 seconds, or until aromatic. Add the remaining can of beans to the mashed bean mixture. Simmer for two minutes, or until thoroughly heated. Turn off the heat and stir in the cheeses, 1/4 cup of cilantro, and 1 lime's juice.
- Get the poblanos ready. Make lengthwise slits in each pepper, leaving the stem whole. In a covered bowl, microwave peppers for 2 1/2 minutes, or until just malleable. Peppers may need to be microwaved in two batches.
- Stuff bean and cheese mixture into peppers. Include corn. Peppers should be baked at 425°F for 30 to 40 minutes, or until they are tender, on a baking sheet.
- Make the tomato salsa in the interim. Mix tomatoes, 1/4 cup cilantro, juice from the remaining lime, and olive oil. Top peppers with tomato salsa and serve.

151. BULGUR VEGETABLE SALAD

Cooking time: 15 mins   **Yield:** 5

Ingredients

- One cup of cooked bulgur
- One cup of finely chopped broccoli
- One cup of coarsely chopped cauliflower
- One red bell pepper
- One scallion, cut (white and green portions)
- Two tablespoons fresh basil leaves
- One lemon's juice and zest
- One tablespoon of olive oil
- Freshly ground black pepper to taste

Instructions

- Combine the bulgur, bell pepper, cauliflower, broccoli, scallion, basil, lemon juice, lemon zest, and olive oil in a big bowl. Add pepper for seasoning.
- After another toss, serve.

152. ROASTED ROOT VEGETABLES

Cooking time: 35 mins   **Yield:** 6

Ingredients

- One cup of chopped turnips

- One cup of chopped rutabaga
- One cup of chopped parsnips
- One tablespoon of extra virgin olive oil
- One teaspoon of finely chopped rosemary
- Freshly ground black pepper, to taste

Instructions

- Set oven temperature to 400°F.
- Combine the parsnips, rutabaga, and turnips in a big bowl along with the rosemary and olive oil. Sprinkle with pepper and arrange in a single layer on a baking sheet.
- Bake, stirring once, for 20 to 25 minutes, or until the veggies are soft and golden.

153. APPLE RICE SALAD

Cooking time: 1 hr   **Yield:** 4

Ingredients

- Two cups of chilled, cooked white short grain rice
- ½ cup thinly sliced celery
- two cups of diced apples (one medium tart and one medium sweet-tart).
- Two teaspoons of shelled, unsalted sunflower seeds
- Half a tsp balsamic vinegar
- One tablespoon of olive oil
- two tsp honey
- Two tsp Dijon mustard

- Two teaspoons of finely crushed orange peel
- one minced garlic clove

Instructions

- In a big bowl, mix cold rice, apple, celery, and sunflower seeds.
- Mix the remaining ingredients together thoroughly with a vigorous whisk in a small bowl.
- Drizzle the rice mixture on top, then gently toss to coat.
- Serve right away or store in the refrigerator for up to 24 hours.

154. CRUNCHY QUINOA SALAD

Cooking time: 20 mins   **Yield:** 8

Ingredients

- 1 cup washed quinoa
- two cups of water
- Five cherry of sliced tomatoes
- a half-cup of diced and seeded cucumbers
- three diced green onions
- half cup of chopped fresh mint
- a half cup of chopped flat-leaf parsley
- two teaspoons chopped fresh lemon juice

- One tablespoon of finely grated lemon zest
- Four tsp olive oil
- Half a head of Boston or Bibb lettuce, cut into cups
- a quarter-cup of grated Parmesan cheese

Instructions

- After well-rinsing the quinoa under cold running water until it's clear, drain it.
- In a skillet over medium-high heat, toast the quinoa for two minutes, tossing often. When it comes to a boil, add two cups of water. For eight to ten minutes, simmer the pan with a lid on and low heat. Allow to cook and use a fork to fluff.
- Add the olive oil, lemon juice, zest, and herbs to the tomatoes, cucumbers, and onions. Stir in the quinoa that has cooled.
- After filling lettuce cups with the mixture, top with grated Parmesan cheese.

155. MEDITERRANEAN CHICKPEA SIDE SALAD

Cooking time: 15 mins   **Yield:** 4

Ingredients

- One (fifteen-and-a-half-oz) can of low-sodium chickpeas
- One cucumber
- ½ cup cherry tomatoes
- Half a red onion
- Feta cheese, two ounces
- One tablespoon of olive oil
- Two tsp red wine vinegar
- One tablespoon of lemon juice
- One tsp of dehydrated oregano
- One tsp dried or fresh parsley

Instructions

- After opening and emptying the chickpea can, rinse it with water.
- Dice the red onion, cucumber, and cherry tomatoes into tiny pieces.
- In a medium-sized bowl, mix together chickpeas, cucumbers, cherry tomatoes, and red onion.
- Finely chop the feta and incorporate it into the bowl.
- Stir together the lemon juice, red wine vinegar, and olive oil and drizzle it over the mixture.
- Add parsley and oregano on top.

156. THAI SALAD WITH CORN

Cooking time: 30 mins   **Yield:** 4-6

Ingredients

- the juice and zest of two limes
- 2 cloves of minced garlic
- about 2-3 teaspoons of Thai sweet chili sauce
- Half a cup of kernels of sweet corn
- Chopped half a red onion
- half a cup of cilantro
- Shredded half a head of cabbage
- half a cup of shredded carrot

Instructions

- In a small bowl, combine lime juice, zest, garlic, and sweet chili sauce; whisk until thoroughly combined. Put aside.
- The remaining ingredients should be combined in a big basin and thoroughly stirred.
- After adding the sauce, toss the vegetable mixture until it is evenly coated.
- Chill for up to 24 hours or serve right away.

157.   COWBOY CAVIAR BEAN & RICE SALAD

Cooking time: 45 mins   **Yield:** 6

Ingredients

- Half a cup cooked corn, fresh or frozen
- three cups boiled rice

- a quarter cup of lime juice
- Half a cup of canola or olive oil
- Two tsp of brown sugar
- One spoonful of mustard dijon
- half a teaspoon of pepper, black
- half a cup of chopped red bell pepper
- 1/2 cup washed and drained low-sodium canned black beans
- One jalapeño, chopped and seeded
- Half a cup of chopped cilantro

Instructions

- When rice and maize are ready, let them cool.
- Lime juice, oil, mustard, brown sugar, and black pepper are combined to form the dressing.
- Combine all other ingredients in a large bowl.
- Drizzle salad with dressing and mix.
- Place in the fridge to chill for one hour.

158.   TORTILLA WRAPS

Cooking time: 22 mins   **Yield:** 2

Ingredients

- two tablespoons of carrots
- Two tsp of green pepper
- one-third cup of cucumber
- 2/3 cup of cooked, unsalted chicken
- Two 6-inch flour tortillas
- Four tsp of softened cream cheese

- one-fourth teaspoon powdered garlic
- 1/4 tsp powdered onion
- 1/3 cup of mixed broccoli slaw

Instructions

- Grate the carrots. Dice the cucumber and green pepper. Cut up chicken.
- Blend onion powder and garlic into cream cheese.
- Over each tortilla, distribute half of the mixture.
- Add the meat and veggies.
- Roll up the wrap, place it in the fridge, or serve right away.

159. EGGPLANT FRENCH FRIES

Cooking time: 30 mins   **Yield:** 6

Ingredients

- One medium eggplant
- One cup of One percent low-fat milk
- Two big eggs
- three quarters cup of cornstarch
- 3/4 cup of breadcrumbs, dry and unseasoned
- Three teaspoons of the dry seasoning and dressing mix for Hidden Valley Original Ranch® salad dressing
- One teaspoon of optional Tabasco® hot sauce

- half a cup of canola oil

Instructions

- Peel and cut the eggplant into 4-inch-long, 3/4-inch sticks. After rinsing, pat dry.
- Blend the eggs and milk thoroughly in a medium-sized bowl, then add the spicy sauce.
- Mix the dry Ranch salad dressing mix, bread crumbs, and cornstarch together in a large, shallow basin.
- Heat the oil in a skillet over high heat.
- After dipping the eggplant sticks into the egg mixture, coat each one with a mixture of bread crumbs.
- Add oil, turning frequently, and cook for three minutes, or until golden brown.
- After draining onto paper towels, serve right away.

160. ASPARAGUS AND TOMATO QUICHE

Cooking time: 50 mins   **Yield:** 4

Ingredients

- One cooking spray that is nonstick
- Ten ounces of asparagus, trimmed and sliced into 2-inch pieces on the diagonal
- Four chopped green onions
- 12 cherry or grape tomatoes, cut in half

- One cup of skim milk
- Four eggs
- Four beaten egg whites
- Two tsp of mustard Dijon
- 1/2 tsp dried thyme or 1 1/2 tsp minced fresh thyme
- A quarter-tsp black pepper
- One-half cup of finely shredded low-fat Colby or cheddar cheese

Instructions

- Set oven temperature to 350°F. Use cooking spray sparingly on a glass pie pan measuring 9 inches.
- Heat the oil in a medium-sized nonstick skillet over medium heat, stirring to coat the bottom. Sauté the green onions and asparagus for 4-5 minutes, or until they are tender. Put the tomatoes and the asparagus mixture in the pie pan.
- Mix all the ingredients except the cheese in a medium-sized bowl. Over the vegetables, pour the mixture. Add a sprinkling of cheese.
- If a knife is placed in the center, it should come out clean after baking for 30 to 35 minutes. After letting the quiche cool for about ten minutes, cut it into four equal pieces.

CHAPTER 10

SNACKS AND SIDE DISHES

161. CUCUMBER AND RADISH SALAD

Cooking time: 12 mins   **Yield:** 4

Ingredients

- 76 grams (⅔ cup) of fresh peas, taken out of their pods
- Thinly slice one medium (312 grams) cucumber
- two Persian cucumbers (124 grams)
- nine large (200 grams) radishes of various sorts
- ¾ cup full-fat Greek yogurt without added sugar or taste
- One tablespoon of lemon juice
- One teaspoon of sumac
- ¼ cup freshly chopped, ribbon-like basil
- Two tablespoons of minced chives

Instructions

- Assign In a small saucepan, combine 2 cups of water and cook over high heat until it boils.
- Give the peas two minutes to blanch. After draining, place the peas in a bowl of ice water to cool.
- Once more, drain and lay away.

- In a bowl, mix together the chilled peas, cucumbers, and radishes.
- In a different, small bowl, combine the yogurt, sumac, and lemon juice.
- Toss in the peas, radishes, cucumbers, and chives along with the yogurt dressing. Blend until well blended.
- Using 4 dishes or plates, divide the salad, putting about ¾ cup of salad in each.

162. BAKED APPLES

Cooking time: 43 mins   **Yield:** 2

Ingredients

- Two medium-sized, tart-sweet apples (Jonagold, Cortland, Braeburn, Honeycrisp, Jonathan)
- Four tsp of brown sugar
- Two teaspoons softened unsalted butter
- One-half teaspoon of cinnamon
- 1/4 tsp ground cloves
- Half a cup of water
- One teaspoon of ground nuts (included in the nutrition analysis but optional)

Instructions

- Turn the oven on to 375°F.

- Peel and core the apples. Give the fillings room to rest at the bottom. If you core the apple all the way through, you can make an apple cup by wrapping aluminum foil over the bottom of the apple.
- Transfer to a baking sheet.
- Mix together the butter, sugar, cloves, cinnamon, and ground nuts (if using).
- Form the mixture into a log form and place half of the mixture into each apple.
- Add water to the pan and bake for 30 to 45 minutes, or until the apples are tender and pricked with a fork.

163. ROASTED BRUSSEL SPROUTS

Cooking time: 50 mins   **Yield:** 8

Ingredients

- Twenty midsize Brussels sprouts
- Three big carrots
- two medium apples
- Two tablespoons of maple syrup
- 1/4 cup of olive oil
- One tsp of cinnamon
- Half a teaspoon of nutmeg
- 1/4 tsp salt

Instructions

- Set oven temperature to 375°F. Apply nonstick cooking spray on a baking sheet.
- After trimming, cut each Brussels sprout in half. After peeling, chop the carrots into 1-inch pieces. Cut the apple into 1/2-inch cubes after covering it.
- Put the apple chunks, carrots, and Brussels sprouts in a big bowl.
- Mix the spices, maple syrup, and olive oil in a small bowl. Mix everything together.
- Toss to coat the apples and veggies in the sauce after adding it to the big bowl. Arrange the components onto the baking sheet. Add the 1/4 teaspoon of salt on top.
- Bake for 30 to 40 minutes, or until Brussels sprouts start to brown and carrots are fork-tender.

164. BAKED TOFU

Cooking time: 50 mins   **Yield:** 5

Ingredients

- 350 grams of extra-firm tofu
- One tablespoon of olive oil
- One tablespoon cornstarch

Tofu With Smoked Paprika (Optional)

- 1/2 tsp paprika smoked
- One-half teaspoon of garlic powder

- One teaspoon ground black pepper

Instructions

- Set oven temperature to 400°F, or 205°C. A few minutes before you're done, prepare the oven by pressing the tofu.
- Unpack the tofu and remove any extra liquid.
- Use paper towels or a fresh, absorbent kitchen towel to cover your tofu.
- Place a hefty object on top of your tofu. Installing the tofu block between two cutting boards and placing canes or mixers on top is my favorite option.
- Lastly, press the tofu for a quarter to a half hour. Draining the tofu is essential, but pressing it is not. You can have crispier baked tofu if you do this.
- Slice the block of tofu into cubes. For uniform cooking, cubes that range in size from 1/2 to 3/4 inches work best.
- Tofu cubes should be oiled and placed in a large mixing dish. Next, if desired, coat them with cornstarch and spices. Spices are not necessary.
- Disperse the tofu cubes onto a parchment paper-lined baking sheet. Bake the cubes in the oven for about thirty minutes, or until they are sufficiently golden to your taste. After 15 minutes of cooking, stir the cubes.

165.   STIR-FRIED GARLIC GREEN BEANS WITH TOASTED ALMONDS

Cooking time: 40 mins   **Yield:** 8

Ingredients

- Three tsp canola oil
- One pound of green beans
- 1/4 cup of almonds, slivered
- two tsp powdered garlic

Instructions

- Turn the heat up to medium-high.
- Toss to evenly coat with oil after adding the green beans.
- Sauté for five minutes.
- Add the garlic powder and almonds.
- Sauté for five minutes.

166.   WHITE BEAN DIP

Cooking time: 35 mins   **Yield:** 8

Ingredients

- Fifteen ounces of reduced-sodium canned white beans
- One clove of garlic
- Half a teaspoon of red pepper flakes
- (1/8 teaspoon dried or 1/4 teaspoon fresh rosemary)
- Three teaspoons of olive oil
- two tsp water
- Five basil leaves

Instructions

- Chop the clove of garlic. Rinse, drain, and put the beans in a strainer.
- Heat two tablespoons of olive oil in a medium-sized pan over low to medium heat. Reduce the heat and add the garlic.
- Add the dried rosemary and red pepper flakes. Stir for about 3 minutes, or until garlic is aromatic.
- Stir in the beans after adding them.
- Once the bean mixture is in a food processor, pulse it. As needed to achieve the desired consistency, add one to two teaspoons of water.
- Take out of the processor and transfer the mixture to a bowl.
- Add the remaining olive oil and basil leaves as garnish.

167.   SWEET POTATO HUMMUS

Cooking time: 1hrs 30mins   **Yield: 4**

Ingredients

- One 15-oz (425-g) can of washed and drained kidney beans
- One 15-oz (425-g) can of washed and drained chickpeas
- 200 g/1 c cooked and peeled orange sweet potato
- Two tablespoons (30 milliliters) tahini

- One teaspoon (5 milliliters) salt that has been iodized
- 1/4 teaspoon (1.2 milliliters) cinnamon
- one garlic clove
- Four to Four and a half tablespoons (67.5–60 mL) of lime juice that has just been squeezed
- 1/2–1 tsp (2.5–5 mL) chili powder to taste (optional) fresh parsley or cilantro

Instructions

- Kidney beans, chickpeas, sweet potato, lime juice, salt, cinnamon, tahini, garlic, and 1/2 tsp (2.5 mL) of chili powder should all be combined in a food processor.
- Blend until smooth, adding 2 tbsp (30 mL) of water gradually to thin the hummus as needed and scraping down the bowl's sides.
- If using, add the fresh parsley or cilantro, and purée just long enough to combine.
- If preferred, add more salt and the final 1/2 tsp (2.5 mL) of chili powder to the dish.

168.   LEMON PEPPER HUMMUS

Cooking time: 35 mins

Ingredients

- 30 ounces (two cans) of canned chickpeas
- one-third cup extra virgin olive oil
- One lemon
- 1 teaspoon of seasoning with lemon pepper and no salt
- one-eighth teaspoon powdered garlic

Instructions

- Place the rinsed and drained chickpeas in a blender or food processor.
- Put one tablespoon of olive oil aside. Add the remaining olive oil, lemon juice, garlic powder, and lemon pepper seasoning to the chickpeas.
- Blend or process until smooth. If needed, thin with 2 to 3 teaspoons of water.
- Transfer to a bowl and drizzle with the tablespoon of olive oil that was set aside.

169.   CRUNCHY VEGGIE CHIPS

Cooking time: 30 mins   **Yield:** 12

Ingredients

- Five bowls of rice cereal that is crunchy.
- Four tsp unsalted butter
- A 12-oz box of marshmallows
- One-third cranberries, dried
- 1/4 cup oats for rapid cooking

- Two tablespoons of tiny chocolate chips
- One-ounce sticks of unsalted pretzels
- 1/4 cup of peanuts, unsalted

Instructions

- Five bowls of rice cereal that is crunchy.
- Four tsp unsalted butter
- A 12-oz box of marshmallows
- Thirty-three cranberries, dried
- 1/4 cup oats for rapid cooking
- Two tablespoons of tiny chocolate chips
- One-ounce sticks of unsalted pretzels
- 1/4 cup of peanuts, unsalted

170.   CUCUMBER DILL CREAM CHEESE BITES

Cooking time: 20 mins   **Yield:** 5

Ingredients

- two medium cucumbers, each measuring around 8 inches
- Eight ounces of room-temperature softened cream cheese
- Greek yogurt with full milk, 4 ounces
- Two tablespoons of dill

Instructions

- Slice cucumbers into pieces that are twenty-five ½ inches thick.

- Using a big spoon or hand mixer, combine cream cheese and Greek yogurt together. Add the dill and stir.
- Spoon one tablespoon of cream cheese equally over four cucumber slices.

171.   SWEET POTATO WEDGES

Cooking time: 1hr 20mins   **Yield:** 1

Ingredients

- Two glasses of unfiltered apple juice or apple cider
- A quarter teaspoon of almond extract
- Cut two large sweet potatoes into eight wedges each.
- Spray vegetable oil

Instructions

for the sauce

- Reduce apple cider to a thick syrupy consistency (approximately ¼ cups) by simmering it in a pot over medium heat for 45 to 1 hour.
- Remain at room temperature after adding the almond essence.

For the Sweet Potatoes

- Set oven temperature to 350°F.
- Make eight wedges out of each potato.
- Sweet potato wedges should be greased before being placed on a

baking pan. Bake for 45 minutes, or until starting to color and become soft. While cooking, turn many times.

- After transferring to a dish, either drizzle the apple cider reduction over the wedges or dip them into it.

172.   EDAMAME DIP

Cooking time: 15 mins   **Yield:** 2

Ingredients

- two cups shelled edamame, around two pounds either frozen or fresh
- One little lemon, squeezed
- One fresh clove smashed or two roasted cloves of garlic
- One rough sliced scallion
- Two tablespoons grated parmesan cheese
- a quarter cup of chopped parsley
- ¼ cup of extra virgin olive oil
- Black pepper that has been freshly ground to taste (optional; not included in nutritional analysis)

Instructions

- In a large saucepan of boiling water, simmer the edamame for five minutes or until they are soft.
- After draining, set aside to cool and reserve ½ cup of the liquid.
- In a food processor or blender, add the edamame, lemon juice, garlic, scallion,

parmesan, and parsley; process until well blended. Add the olive oil gradually while the machine is running and process until smooth.

- Add pepper to taste, if desired. To get the right consistency, add a few tablespoons of cooking liquid at a time, as needed.
- Keep chilled in a sealed receptacle.

173.   KIDNEY-FRIENDLY GUACAMOLE

Cooking time: 5 mins   **Yield:** 6

Ingredients

- One large, soft avocado
- one squeezed lime
- two minced garlic cloves
- 1/4 cup finely chopped onions
- one chopped jalapeño
- 1/4 cup finely chopped fresh cilantro
- One pinch of salt

Instructions

- In a bowl, mix the avocado and lime juice. Using a fork, mash to the desired consistency.
- Stir in the remaining components. Toss to blend. Have fun!

174.   HEALTHY CORN FRITTERS

Cooking time: 30 mins   **Yield:** 4

Ingredients

- 3 cups of fresh or frozen corn, chopped off the cob
- Half a cup of all-purpose flour
- Two teaspoons of sugar
- One-fourth teaspoon baking soda
- 1/4 tsp powdered garlic
- 1½ teaspoon powdered onion
- Two cayenne pepper dashes
- 1/8 teaspoon salt
- 1/4 teaspoon ground pepper
- One lightly beaten egg
- one-third cup low-fat milk
- One tablespoon of canola oil

Instructions

- In a sizable mixing bowl, mix together corn, flour, sugar, baking soda, spices, salt, and pepper. Mix until well blended.
- Pour in the milk and the egg. Stir just until everything is incorporated.
- In a skillet over medium heat, heat the oil.
- To make each fritter, drop 1/4 cup of the batter into a hot skillet. To make the fritters slightly thinner (approximately 1/4 inch thick), slightly press down on the batter. Cook for 3–5 minutes on

each side, or until well cooked and browned.

- If preferred, garnish with a green onion or any of the suggested toppings. Have fun!

175.   FRENCH FRIES MADE WITH ZUCCHINI

Cooking time: 45 mins   **Yield:** 6

Ingredients

- two medium-sized zucchini
- One cup of 1% nonfat milk
- Two big eggs
- one-third cup cornstarch
- 3/4 cup of breadcrumbs, dry and unseasoned
- three dry tablespoons Original Ranch® Salad Dressing and Seasoning Mix from Hidden Valley
- One teaspoon of optional Tabasco® hot sauce
- half a cup of canola oil

Instructions

- Peel and cut the zucchini into 4-inch-long, 3/4-inch sticks. After rinsing, pat dry the zucchini.
- Blend the eggs and milk thoroughly in a medium-sized bowl, then add the spicy sauce.
- Mix the dry Ranch salad dressing mix, bread crumbs, and cornstarch together in a large, shallow basin.
- Heat the oil in a skillet over high heat.
- After dipping zucchini sticks into the egg mixture, coat each one with a coating of bread crumbs.
- Add oil, turning frequently, and cook for three minutes, or until golden brown.
- After draining onto paper towels, serve right away.

CHAPTER 11

DESSERT RECIPES

176. FRUIT CRISPIES

Cooking time: 60 mins **Yield:** 1

Ingredients

- One can (eighteen ounces) of drained peaches in their own juice
- one tsp lemon juice
- Half a cup of brown sugar
- 1/4 cup of white flour
- 3/4 cup of oats
- One-half teaspoon of cinnamon
- half a teaspoon of nutmeg
- ¼ stick unsalted chilled butter

Instructions

- Set the oven's temperature to 350°F.
- Place the peaches in a muffin tray that has been greased, then drizzle with lemon juice.
- Mix the spices, flour, oats, and brown sugar together.
- Until the mixture resembles wet sand, cut in butter.
- Dredge in the fruit mixture.
- Bake for bubbling and browned, 25 to 30 minutes.
- Warm up and serve.

177. KETO BROWNIE

Cooking time: 40 mins **Yield:** 8

Ingredients

- ½ cup butter without salt
- ¼ cup of strongly brewed coffee
- One cup of almond flour
- ½ cup chocolate powder, unsweetened
- Half a teaspoon of salt
- ¾ cup granulated monk fruit sweetener
- Three big, room-temperature eggs
- One tsp vanilla essence

Instructions

- Set the oven's temperature to 175°C/350°F. Using parchment paper, line an 8-inch square pan.
- In a small saucepan set over low to medium heat, add the butter.
- Once melted, heat the butter until it smells nutty and turns golden brown. Stir continuously.
- Take the browned butter saucepan off of the burner. It is essential to remove the butter from the heat source because it is simple for the combination to burn on residual burner heat.
- Blend the brewed espresso with the butter that has browned. You can have

hot or cold espresso. Refrigerate the mixture for a while.

- Mix the almond flour, cocoa powder, salt, and monk fruit in a medium-sized bowl.
- Whisk together the eggs and vanilla extract in another medium-sized basin.
- Make sure the mixture of browned butter and cools almost completely before adding the eggs and vanilla. Note: Give the browned butter plenty of time to cool down because too much heat will cause the eggs to fry.
- Stir the wet ingredients (browned butter and egg) into the dry ingredients (almond flour, cocoa, salt, and monk fruit).
- Toss to combine the keto brownie batter and stir until well combined.
- Transfer the keto brownie mixture into the 8-inch pan that has been preheated.
- In a preheated oven, bake the keto brownies for 20 minutes. When a toothpick inserted into the brownies comes out with very few crumbs, it is done. After 20 minutes, if the toothpick is still wet, extend the duration by 5 minutes at a time.
- After baking, let the keto brownies cool fully in the pan before slicing, serving, and savoring.
- Adding sugar-free whipped cream or keto-friendly ice cream on top is optional!

178.   POOR MAN'S CAKE

Cooking time: 60 mins   **Yield:** 24

Ingredients

- Three cups of white all-purpose flour
- two cups of sugar
- half a cup cocoa
- Half a teaspoon each of salt and baking soda
- two tsp of vinegar
- three-quarter cup of vegetable oil
- two tsp vanilla
- two glasses of cold water

Instructions

- Set oven temperature to 350°F.
- In a 9 x 13-inch ungreased baking pan, combine the first 5 ingredients.
- In the dry ingredients, create three holes.
- Fill one hole with two teaspoons of vinegar.
- Fill the second hole with 3/4 cup of oil.
- Add two tsp of vanilla extract to the third opening.
- Mix in two glasses of cold water.
- When a toothpick put into the center comes out clean, bake for 30 to 45 minutes.

179.   APPLE PIE

Cooking time: 2 hrs   **Yield:** 8

Ingredients

- Six medium-sized apples
- 1/2 cup of sugar, granulated
- one tsp finely ground cinnamon
- six tsp butter
- 2-2/3 cups flour for all purposes
- One cup of shortening
- six tsp water

Instructions

- Set oven temperature to 425°F.
- Slice, core, and peel apples.
- Combine apple slices, sugar, and cinnamon in a large bowl. Put a cover on and leave it alone.
- Using a pastry blender, mix the shortening into the flour in a large, separate basin. One spoonful at a time, add cold water and stir until dough comes together into a ball. If not, create a ball with your hands.
- Using a rolling pin and extra flour as needed, divide the dough in two and flatten out one portion. Put into a 9-inch pie pan.
- After stirring, transfer the apple pie filling into the pie crust.
- Distribute the butter evenly around the pie filling using pats measuring one tablespoon.
- Roll out your remaining half of dough. Make sure the pie's edges are covered when you place it on top of the apple pie filling.
- Cut four 1" slits around the top of the pie crust with a sharp knife to allow air to escape while baking.
- Pie should be baked on a jelly roll pan to collect any juice that may leak while baking.
- Bake until the crust is golden brown, about 50 to 60 minutes.

180.   BUTTERSCOTCH BARS

Cooking time: 40 mins   **Yield:** 18

Ingredients

- 1/2 cup of flour for all purposes
- One tsp baking powder
- Half a teaspoon of salt
- half a cup of butter without salt
- Two cups of densely packed brown sugar
- Two big eggs
- One tsp vanilla essence

Instructions

- Set oven temperature to 350°F. Apply nonstick cooking spray to a 9 x 13-inch baking pan.
- Mix the flour, baking powder, and salt in a medium-sized bowl.

- In a bowl that is microwave-safe, melt the butter. Brown sugar should be added and stirred until dissolved. Add the vanilla and eggs and stir.
- Add the flour mixture and stir.
- After filling the baking pan with batter, bake the bars for 30 minutes, or until the center of the bars is set.
- While the bars are still warm, cut into 18 squares.

181.   YELLOW CAKE

Cooking time: 15 mins   **Yield:** 6

Ingredients

- One packet of flavorless gelatin
- Three cups of frozen or fresh strawberries
- Ten tablespoons of sugar, granulated
- Pasteurized egg whites, 3/4 cup
- One cup of whipped topping

Instructions

- To dissolve the gelatin, combine 1 tablespoon of water with the gelatin in a small bowl and microwave for 10 to 15 seconds. After stirring, put away.
- Handle clean and dehulled strawberries. Three sliced strawberries should be set aside for garnish.
- In a food processor, purée the berries. Transfer the purée into a bowl and whisk in the gelatin. Add enough sugar

to taste between two and four tablespoons. Put aside.
- Transfer egg whites to a sanitized mixing bowl. Beat until tender peaks form.
- Six tablespoons of sugar should be added gradually to egg whites as they are beating until firm and glossy.
- Mix the egg whites with the strawberry puree by folding. Transfer the mixture to a dessert glass or glass bowl and refrigerate.
- Serve the mousse with whipped topping on top and strawberry slices as a garnish right before serving.

182.   MARGARITA FREEZER PIE

Cooking time: 6hrs 50mins   **Yield:** 10

Ingredients

- Five cups of vanilla bean low-fat ice cream
- Six ounces of concentrated frozen limeade
- Two new limes
- One to two drops of optional green food coloring
- Crust of one graham cracker

Instructions

- Thaw the limeade concentrate and set the ice cream out to soften. Measure out two tablespoons of lime peel to add to the pie mixture after zesting it. Zest the lime, juice it, and measure out 1 tablespoon.

- In a big bowl, mix the softened ice cream, limeade, juice, and zest. Blend thoroughly by stirring.
- Fill the graham cracker crust with filling. Once solid, cover and freeze.
- Divide pie into ten portions. Add a fresh lime slice as a garnish to each slice.

183.   PINEAPPLE ANGEL CAKE

Cooking time: 30 mins   **Yield:** 12

Ingredients

- One package of angel food cake mix
- 20 ounces of canned crushed pineapple
- 8-ounces of juice pack Thawed Cool Whip® frozen dessert topping

Instructions

- Set oven temperature to 350°F.
- Using a mixer, thoroughly mix and beat in the whole can of undrained pineapple. Add the dry cake mix.
- Fill a 9" by 13" cake pan that hasn't been greased with ingredients. Bake until the tops are gently browned, 25 to 30 minutes.
- Let cool fully.

- Use whipped topping without dairy to frost. Keep refrigerated.

184.   FRUIT PIZZA

Cooking time: 2 hrs   **Yield:** 12

Ingredients

- One medium apple
- two and a half teaspoons lemon juice
- Twenty grapes
- Four medium-sized strawberries
- half a cup of sugar
- One cup of pineapple juice
- two tsp cornstarch
- One roll of frozen sugar cookie dough
- Whipped cream cheese (12 ounces)

Instructions

- Turn the oven on to 325°F.
- Apple core and thinly slice. Mix 1/2 tsp lemon juice with the apple pieces. Cut strawberries into slices and cut grapes in half.
- Stir together cornstarch, sugar, pineapple juice, and the remaining lemon juice over medium heat until thickened.
- Cut cookie dough into 1/4-inch pieces. Arrange closely on a pizza pan that has been coated with nonstick cooking spray.

- Bake according to the package's instructions or until brown, at 325° F. Place aside to cool fully.
- On the chilled cookie shell, spread cream cheese.
- Place sliced fruit on top of the cream cheese. To make a masterpiece, use your imagination!
- Transfer the fruit to a chilled pineapple glaze and store in the refrigerator for a few hours before serving.

185. GINGERBREAD APPLE COBBLER

Cooking time: 50 mins   **Yield:** 8

Ingredients

- Four cups of apples
- one-third cup of brown sugar
- One tablespoon of lemon juice
- Three-quarter teaspoon cinnamon
- One cup of water
- One tablespoon cider vinegar
- Two tablespoons cornstarch
- Seven tsp low-fat milk
- one-fourth cup sugar
- One egg
- Half a cup of light molasses
- two tsp of corn syrup
- Two tsp of oil
- One cup of flour for all purposes
- One-half tsp baking soda

- One-half tsp baking powder
- Half a teaspoon of ginger powder
- Half a cup of whipped cream for garnish

Instructions

- Set oven temperature to 350°F.
- Cut and peel the apples. In a medium saucepan, combine apples, brown sugar, lemon juice, 1 cup water, and 1/2 teaspoon cinnamon. Cook the apples covered until they are soft.
- Stir cornstarch into hot apple sauce after combining it with 1 tablespoon of water. Cooking should be continued until thickened. Transfer the apple mixture to a 1-1/2-quart casserole and keep it covered.
- Stir in 1 tablespoon of vinegar with milk. Put aside.
- Beat together oil, molasses, corn syrup, egg, milk mixture, and sugar.
- Mix the flour, baking powder, baking soda, ginger, and the remaining 1/4 teaspoon of cinnamon in a different basin. Beat until smooth after adding to the beaten egg and milk mixture.
- Cover the apples in the casserole with the gingerbread mixture. For thirty minutes, bake.
- Serve warm, garnished with 1 tablespoon of whipped cream or dessert topping.

186. APPLE CRISP

Cooking time: 2 hrs   **Yield:** 16

Ingredients

- Six medium-sized apples
- two tsp of cinnamon
- 2-1/3 cups of sugar
- Three cups of white all-purpose flour
- One cup of canola oil
- Four big eggs
- one-fourth cup orange juice
- One-third tsp baking powder
- Two and a half teaspoons of vanilla extract

Instructions

- Set oven temperature to 350°F.
- Apply non-stick cooking spray to the tube pan.
- Cut apples into chunks or slices after peeling and cored.
- Add 1/3 cup sugar and cinnamon together. Add apple and stir; put aside.
- The remaining ingredients should be combined in a bowl and smoothed out with an electric mixer.
- In a prepared tube pan, layer half of the cake batter, followed by the apple, and then the remaining cake batter.
- Bake for seventy-five minutes, or until the toothpick inserted in the center comes out clean, or until golden brown.

187. BLUEBERRY PEACH CRISP

Cooking time: 55 mins   **Yield:** 10

Ingredients

- Seven medium-sized peaches
- One cup of blueberries
- 1/4 cup of sugar, granulated
- One tablespoon of lemon juice
- 3/4 cup of flour for all purposes
- 3/4 cup of dense brown sugar
- half a cup of butter

Instructions

- Warm the oven up to 375°F.
- Pit peaches and cut them into 3/4-inch slices.
- Coat the 12" x 9" baking dish with cooking spray. Put the blueberries and peach slices on a plate.
- Scatter lemon juice and sugar on top of the fruit.
- In a bowl, combine the flour and brown sugar. Crumble the butter into the flour and sugar mixture using two knives or a pastry blender. Over the fruit, scatter crumbs.
- Bake for a minimum of 45 minutes, or until the crumbs are toasted and the fruit is tender.
- Heat or serve at room temperature.

188. WARM BREAD PUDDING

Cooking time: 1hr 25mins   **Yield:** 6

Ingredients

- Two big eggs
- two white eggs
- 1.5 cups almond milk
- One teaspoon vanilla and two teaspoons honey
- One teaspoon of rum extract or two teaspoons of rum
- Four pieces of raisin bread

Instructions

- Set the oven temperature to 325° F.
- Apply nonstick cooking spray to an 8-inch circular baking dish.
- Beat the egg whites and eggs together in a large mixing basin until frothy. Stir in rum or rum extract, honey, vanilla, and almond milk.
- Cube the bread and add it to the egg mixture. Fill the baking dish with prepared mixture.
- When a knife inserted in the center comes out clean, bake for 35 to 40 minutes.
- Spoon warm pudding into dessert bowls to serve.

189. PALACSINTA (DESSERT PANCAKES)

Cooking time: 30 mins   **Yield:** 16

Ingredients

- four cups cottage cheese without fat
- Two cups of white all-purpose flour
- Six tablespoons sugar, separated
- one-sixteenth teaspoon of salt
- two eggs
- Two cups of liquid nondairy creamer
- Nonstick cooking spray
- half a cup of raisins
- One spoonful of powdered sugar and 1/4 teaspoon of vanilla extract

Instructions

- Put the cottage cheese onto a cheesecloth and roll it into a ball to produce the filling. Transfer to a colander, set the colander inside a mixing bowl, and, for safety's sake, refrigerate. Let the liquid settle for a minimum of two hours.
- Combine flour, salt, and 1 tablespoon sugar.
- After gently beating the eggs in another bowl, mix in the non-dairy creamer.
- Whisk the flour mixture into the egg mixture until a thin, homogeneous batter forms. Give the batter one hour to rest.

- Apply non-stick cooking spray and preheat an 8-inch omelet pan.
- Once bubbles form in the center of the 1/4 cup of batter, turn the pan over.
- When you're ready to assemble, stack the pancakes onto a dinner plate and keep warm in the oven.
- Stir together the drained cottage cheese, raisins, vanilla, and five tablespoons of sugar.
- After adding 1/4 cup of filling to each palacsinta, roll it up. Before serving, dust with powdered sugar.

190. HOME-STYLE VANILLA ICE CREAM

Cooking time: 2hrs 30mins   **Yield:** 8

Ingredients

- One cup of low-fat egg product
- half a cup of sugar
- Two cups of non dairy liquid creamer
- One tablespoon of vanilla extract
- rock salt and ice (for an ice cream maker machine)

Instructions

- In a microwaveable 1-quart bowl, mix egg product and sugar together until thoroughly combined.
- After mixing in a non-dairy creamer, microwave the mixture for one minute, or until it thickens.
- Take off the heat. Add vanilla when it has cooled.
- Transfer the mixture into the ice cream maker's central container.
- Around the container, alternate layers of ice and rock salt until the bucket is full.
- Process in accordance with your specific ice cream machine's manufacturer's recommendations.

Chapter 12

Beverages and Smoothies

191. Blueberry Bliss Smoothie

Yield: 2

Ingredients

- half a cup of frozen or boiled cauliflower
- half a cup of frozen blueberries or mixed berries two spoonful (three tablespoons) Powdered beneprotein
- One tablespoon honey
- One-half teaspoon of cinnamon
- ½ cup almond milk without sugar
- Half a cup of water

Instructions

- Steam cauliflower for 5 to 7 minutes, or until it becomes soft.
- After transferring the cauliflower to a baking dish, freeze it for at least two hours.
- Put all ingredients in a blender and process until smooth on high speed.

192. Easy Pineapple Protein Smoothie

Yield: 1

Ingredients

- 3/4 cup sorbet or sherbet made of pineapple
- One scoop of protein powdered vanilla whey
- half a cup of water
- Two ice cubes, if desired

Instructions

- Pour water, whey protein powder, and pineapple sherbet into a blender (ice cubes optional).
- Blend for 30 to 45 seconds right away.

193. Mixed Berry Protein Smoothie

Yield: 2

Ingredients

- Four ounces of icy water
- 1 cup mixed berries, either fresh or frozen
- Two cubes of ice
- One teaspoon of any berry-flavored Crystal Light® liquid flavor enhancer drops
- Half a cup of whipped cream topping
- Whey protein powder, two scoops

Instructions

- Pour water, ice cubes, frozen berries, and liquid flavor enhancer drops into a blender. Mix thoroughly and blend until slushy.
- Mix in the whipped topping thoroughly.
- Put some protein powder in. Mix thoroughly.
- Split into two portions, and either eat one immediately away or freeze and reheat at a later time.

194.   PEACH HIGH-PROTEIN FRUIT SMOOTHIE

Yield: 1

Ingredients

- Half a cup of ice
- Two teaspoons of powdered egg whites, or Just Whites®
- three-quarter cup of fresh peaches
- One spoonful of sugar

Instructions

- Blend the peaches in the blender until they are smooth.
- Blend all the ingredients until they are smooth after adding them.

195.   APPLE CINNAMON SMOOTHIE

Yield: 2

Ingredients

- One cup of unsweetened applesauce without additional vitamin C
- Four tablespoons of canola oil
- Half a cup of apple cider
- ⅓ cup instant or normal oatmeal
- 1/4 tsp each of vanilla extract
- 1/4 teaspoon of cinnamon
- One tablespoon of cream cheese

Instructions

- This smoothie tastes really light. For optimal results, all ingredients (except from the canola/vegetable oil) must be kept cool before combining.
- In the blender, combine all the ingredients and process for 4 minutes, or until smooth. To make it simpler for the oats to blend in, I suggest adding the applesauce first. If desired, you can put a little more cinnamon on top. If you use gluten-free oats, the recipe is also gluten-free.

196.   COCO COFFEE FRAPPE

Yield: 2

Ingredients

- Three-quarter cup of strong brewed coffee at room temperature
- One-and-a-quarter cup of ice
- Half a cup of coconut milk
- Two tsp of maple syrup
- One-quarter teaspoon of cinnamon

Instructions

- Fill the blender with all of the ingredients.
- In a regular blender, blend for roughly one minute, or until very frothy.
- Transfer to two glasses.
- Garnish with extra ice and a dash of cinnamon, if desired.

197.   TAMARIND DRINK

Yield: 10

Ingredients

- One-pound pods of tamarind
- Half a cup of divided sugar
- two quarts of water
- Two-inch ginger ice cubes, weighing six grams

Instructions

- Split open the tamarind shells and remove the pulp. Cut the strings.
- Boil three cups of water.
- After peeling the pods, put them in a basin and pour the three cups of boiling water over them. Allow to stand for the entire night.
- To aid in the pulp's separation from the seeds, whisk the tamarind pod solution in the bowl. Process on low power in a mixer, if desired. Throw away the seeds.
- Press the pulp with a spoon or spatula to strain it through a sieve.
- Pour the tamarind paste through a strainer into a gallon jug. To make two quarts of tamarind juice, add the remaining one quart and one cup of water.
- To taste, dissolve sugar in the juice.
- Grate in the ginger and thoroughly mix in.
- Put it in the fridge for a minimum of 60 minutes.
- Serve it with cubes of ice.

198.   STRAWBERRY HIGH-PROTEIN FRUIT SMOOTHIE

Yield: 1

Ingredients

- three-quarter cup of raw strawberries
- half a cup of pasteurized liquid egg whites
- Half a cup of ice
- One spoonful of sugar

Instructions

- In a blender, combine the strawberries and process until smooth.
- Blend all the ingredients until they are smooth after adding them.

199. PAPAYA SMOOTHIE

Yield: 1

Ingredients

- three ounces of small-cut, chopped papaya
- ½ cup of unsweetened oat or almond milk
- One tsp honey
- ½ teaspoon grated fresh ginger
- Lime juice, two tablespoons
- Two cubes of ice

Instructions

- In a blender, combine the papaya, milk, honey, lime, and ginger.
- Process for 15 seconds at a medium speed.
- Include the ice cubes.
- To get smooth, process at high speed for about 30 seconds; extend if needed.

- Pour into glasses and savor!

200. TRIPLE BERRY SMOOTHIE

Yield: 1

Ingredients

- Half a cup of strawberries
- A quarter cup of raspberries
- One-quarter cup of blackberries
- Half cup of Almond milk
- Handful of baby spinach

Instructions

- Incorporate the blackberries, raspberries, strawberries, and a small handful of baby spinach into the blender.
- Pour the two cups of almond or coconut milk into the mixture.
- Blend until smooth and achieve the desired texture of a smoothie!
- Smoothie should be served in a glass with extra fresh sliced strawberries as a garnish. All set to sip!

CHAPTER 13

DINING OUT AND SOCIALIZING

Going out to eat at a great restaurant, or obtaining take-out or delivery to enjoy at home for movie night, is something that many of us enjoy and anticipate. During the holiday season, you may receive more invitations to eat out than normal, as well as invites to holiday parties and events where food is the focus.

Living with chronic kidney disease (CKD) does not require you to stay at home and lose out on activities; all you need to do is plan ahead of time. This chapter will teach you how to keep your sodium, protein, potassium, and phosphorus levels under control while having fun. Not only that, but this chapter will assist you decide what to order when you visit your favorite Italian or Asian restaurant. Let us get you ready to go out and have fun!

EATING OUT IN DIFFERENT RESTAURANTS

Dining out at restaurants can be tough if you have CKD. If you have a favorite restaurant, ask the manager for a copy of the menu to go to your unit dietician, who will assist you in making informed decisions.

ITALIAN RESTAURANTS

Italy is known for its high phosphorus, potassium, and sodium content, including pizza. But don't worry. There are still some choices for you. Obviously, pizza is not particularly dialysis-friendly. If you do order it on occasion, I recommend a thin crust with pesto, onion, and garlic; if you enjoy pineapple, that may be a fun addition. You may also choose a vegetarian pizza (low on cheese, no tomatoes, sun-dried tomatoes), which would avoid processed salty meats such as pepperoni and sausage. Have a couple of slices and pair them with a salad.

Some foods to look out for:

- Antipasti starter platters include cheese, olives, and cured salty meats.

- Lasagna, cannelloni, ravioli, and tortellini (all loaded with cheese and tomato sauce).
- Spaghetti/pasta with marinara, Napoletana, Bolognese, cacciatore, arrabbiata sauce (all tomato-based).
- Carbonara (pancetta, egg yolks, heavy cream, cheese) and Alfredo pasta (cream, Parmesan cheese).
- Eggplant Parmesan

Your best bets:

- Sourdough bread dipped in olive oil and balsamic vinegar (great with crushed garlic!).
- Mixed green salad (without tomatoes). Request no salad dressing and instead offer olive oil and balsamic vinegar on the side to limit sodium levels and add your own salt-free spice.
- Pesto pasta (no extra parmesan).
- Capellini or angel hair pasta with olive oil, garlic, and basil, but instead of pomodoro (fresh tomatoes), request zucchini, bell pepper, or eggplant, with the option of adding shrimp or a meat of your choosing.
- Pasta primavera (without tomatoes).
- Fresh fish or seafood.
- Chicken Piccata with Lemon Butter Sauce

ASIAN RESTAURANTS

These are difficult places to eat due to the high sodium level. Chinese restaurants are the most difficult due to the enormous amount of combined meals with soy, hoisin, and sweet and sour sauces. They all include salt and/or MSG. Thai cuisine is known for its abundance of spices and low salt content; sauces are frequently available on request. Japanese eateries will also provide more spicy meals and use less sodium. Try these options:

Chinese

Chinese culinary essentials consist of rice, noodles, vegetables, beef, poultry, eggs, and tofu. Many people like this option when eating out, however, it is generally rich in sodium, bad fats, and sugar, and it frequently contains MSG (monosodium glutamate) as a taste enhancer. When you place your order, ask if they can prepare your food without soy sauce, fish sauce, or MSG. *Some foods to look out for:*

- I'd avoid all soups. They are quite high in sodium.

- Fried Egg Rolls.
- Fried rice and noodles.
- General Tso's/orange/sweet and sour chicken and sweet and sour pork (deep-fried meat coated in syrupy sauce)
- Barbecue spare ribs. This appears innocent, but it is a high-fat, salt, and sugar meal.
- Kung Pao chicken. High in salt and contains peanuts.

Your best bet:

- Dim sum steamed dumplings.
- Steamed rice. Ask for brown rice. It provides more fiber and reduces blood sugar spikes.
- Buddha's Delight (stir-fried vegetables and tofu). You can order the steamed version without the sauce. Use coconut aminos instead!
- Chop Suey (a stir-fried dish made from pork, eggs, and vegetables). Order with chicken or shrimp with brown rice.
- Egg Foo Young. Ask for it to be lightly fried.
- Moo goo gai pan (chicken and vegetable stir-fry). Request sauce on the side.
- Chicken or beef with broccoli. Light on the sauce (or serve on the side).

Thai

I enjoy a good Thai meal, but like Chinese food, it is typically filled with soy sauce, fish sauce, MSG, and harmful oils. Regardless, you can choose healthier solutions for yourself. *Some foods to look out for:*

- Deep-fried egg rolls and wontons
- All soups
- Papaya salad (rich in potassium)
- Thai curries (red, green, and yellow). They are high in sodium and use canned coconut milk as a basis, which is extremely high in potassium.
- Thai Fried Rice. Opt for the healthier steamed version.
- Gluay kaeg (fried banana treat) and fried ice cream
- Thai iced tea (made from sweetened condensed milk)

Your best bets are:

- Fresh spring/summer rolls. I love these! They are frequently served with peanut and sweet sauce, so don't overdo the dipping. Avoid fried foods.

- Steamed rice. If you're feeling energetic, try brown rice.
- Larb chicken salad. Ask if it can be done without fish sauce.
- Pad Thai noodles can be prepared with shrimp, chicken, or tofu. Hold the peanuts and request a mild oil and side sauce (which contains fish sauce). You can also have a side of steamed vegetables.
- Beef & broccoli
- Steamed fish and veggies.

Japanese

White rice, salmon, fresh and pickled vegetables, seaweed, and miso-flavored tofu are staples of the traditional Japanese diet. Sushi is a traditional cuisine that consists of raw fish rolled up with vinegared rice, seaweed, and veggies. However, sushi can be made without using raw fish. Eating Japanese food is another great opportunity to bring your coconut aminos along for a lower-sodium dipping sauce.

After a transplant, you must avoid raw fish (sashimi, raw fish sushi) since your immune system will be inhibited. Foods that are more likely to cause foodborne illness or parasite infections should be avoided. Some argue that dialysis patients should avoid eating raw fish for the same reasons, although this is not a hard and fast rule.

Some foods to look out for:

- Wasabi (rich in sodium, but also includes potassium).
- Edamame is an immature soybeans in pods that are typically served steamed with salt. High in potassium.
- Ramen, soups (high salt content).
- Miso-based dressings and soups.
- Natto (a fermented soybean-based morning meal). Potassium levels are very high.
- Seaweed salad (rich in sodium, potassium, and MSG).
- Avoid sushi rolls containing too much sauce, avocado, nuts, or yam.

Your best bets:

- Gyoza are tiny dumplings filled with meat and veggies. Request that they be steamed without sauce.
- Onigiri rice balls are typically packed with meat or veggies. Ask for no black sesame seeds.
- California roll (no avocado) and other rolls including cooked eel, shrimp, or crab.

- Yakitori (grilled chicken skewers).
- bento boxes. Rice, fish, or meat are frequently served with pickled veggies. Watch your portions because they may contain more sodium.
- Tempura. It's not particularly nutritious because it's deep-fried in a light batter (typically vegetables, shrimp, and prawns), so treat yourself!
- Hibachi or teppanyaki-style grilling (noodles, veggies, pork, fish, and tofu). Pay attention to the sauce.

Note: Avoid soups in all Asian restaurants, as well as most other restaurants. They are all made from canned or dried stock, have a high salt level, and add more fluid to your regular intake. Also, avoid noodles and broth-based dishes because they are rather salty.

MEXICAN

Who does not love tacos? I enjoy Mexican food too, but it can be rich in salt, potassium, and phosphorus. *Some foods to look out for:*

- Salted fried tortilla chips. So addictive and high in salt and bad fats. If you're like me and can't stop at just a handful, avoid it.
- salsas and tomato-based sauces.
- Chili en carne: kidney beans, beef, and tomato sauce.
- Menu items include quesadillas, cheese enchiladas, and chile relleno. Tomales are reserved for special occasions.
- Guacamole
- Refried beans.
- Nachos

What's left to eat, right? Many delicious foods, but not so kidney-friendly. *Your best bets:*

- Tacos. Choose from beef, chicken, fish, shrimp, or vegetarian tacos (with black or pinto beans), cilantro, lettuce/cabbage, onions, and sour cream. This is an excellent moment to add your salt-free spicy sauce!
- Fajitas. Beef or chicken. They are frequently served with sautéed onions and bell peppers, which are low in potassium. You can make a veggie fajita by omitting the meat and substituting mushrooms and zucchini. Choose a side of rice instead of beans.

161

- Chicken or beef enchiladas with a mild green sauce.

Burritos made using flour tortillas can contain high levels of salt and phosphorus. When you add higher salt meats like shredded carnitas and chorizo, you'll consume the majority of your daily sodium intake just from the tortilla. Instead, make chicken or beef burritos with rice, lettuce/cabbage, onions, and your own no-salt spicy sauce.

For a fun twist, try adding a small bit of tomatillo salsa. If your potassium levels are under control and you're craving avocado, instead of guacamole, request a small side of sliced avocado and add a couple to your plate. A tiny quantity is fine, but more than that can significantly elevate your potassium levels.

INDIAN

Indian cuisine features classic spices including curry, turmeric, ginger, chiles, cumin, and coriander. Rice, roti (whole wheat unleavened flatbread) naan (leavened flatbread), and dal (a lentil stew) are all staple foods. This can be eaten with a vegetable or a meat/chicken/seafood dish, along with a yogurt sauce (raita), pickles, chutneys, and other relish condiments. I enjoy a delicious Indian dish, but they are often rich in sodium and potassium. *Here are some foods to look out for:*

- Dal (lentil soup)
- Chicken tikka masala (tomato yogurt sauce).
- Malai kofta (vegetarian "meatballs" prepared from potato, almonds, paneer cheese, and served in a creamy tomato/nut sauce)
- Chole chickpea curry. Most curries will be heavy in salt and potassium.
- Palak paneer (a dish made of spinach and Indian cottage cheese)
- Chaat (a crispy snack item typically with a fried cracker and topped with potatoes, tomatoes, chickpeas, yogurt, and chutney)
- Rajma (kidney beans in rich gravy)
- Lassi (sweet yogurt drink with milk and fruit)

Your best bets:

- Naan and Roti flatbread
- Meat Samosas are deep-fried pastries stuffed with meat or veggies. The vegetable version contains potatoes and lentils, therefore it is best avoided.

162

- Momos are steamed dumplings filled with tandoori chicken, pork, fish, or eggplant. Prepared by roasting in a clay oven.
- Biryani is a spiced rice meal with meat, while meat kebabs are another option.
- Gobi matar (cauliflower with peas). Order dry, without the masala sauce.

GREEK

I adore Greece, its history, and its food! Greek cuisine consists of olive oil (the major component in most meals), olives, feta cheese, Greek honey, fruits, legumes, vegetables, fresh herbs, yogurt, fish/seafood, and lamb. The good news is that there are numerous healthy options for dialysis sufferers! *Some foods to look out for:*

- Moussaka is a layered casserole with tomato sauce covered with bechamel.
- Pastitsio is a baked meal similar to lasagna that consists of layers of pasta, tomato sauce, and ground meat, topped with bechamel.
- Spanakopita is a spinach pie made with feta cheese, eggs, and herbs wrapped in filo dough.
- Saganaki is fried cheese seasoned with salt. High in sodium and phosphorus.

Your best bets:

- Greek salad. This comprises feta cheese, onion, cucumber, and bell pepper. Request no tomatoes and just olive oil instead of dressing.
- Dolma/dolmades are grape leaves loaded with rice, herbs, veggies, or meat. Squeeze some lemon juice on top for an extra taste.
- Hummus (made with ground chickpeas and tahini). Portion sizes should be limited because of the high salt and potassium content.
- Pita bread. As with all bread, it will increase your sodium intake, but a small amount with hummus is acceptable.
- Tabouli (Tabouleh). A salad made of bulgar wheat, parsley, and a tiny amount of tomatoes, mint, and onion, dressed with olive oil and lemon juice.
- Gyros are a popular street snack. Rotisserie meat (typically lamb) in a pita with onions, lettuce, tomato, and tzatziki. It may contain significant amounts of sodium and potassium. Request no tomatoes and tzatziki sauce on the side.
- Souvlaki or kebabs. Grilled meat is frequently eaten straight off the skewer. Traditionally served with pita, vegetables, and tzatziki on the side.

- Fresh fish.
- Couscous (pasta made from semolina and wheat flour). A good source of fiber and protein.

When you eat out, your sodium intake will be higher than if you ate at home. Remember to meet your dietary and fluid requirements. Use chewing gum, hard candy, breath sprays, and other thirst suppressants to keep your weight gain to less than 5% of your dry weight. If you eat a lot of potassium-rich foods, be extra cautious. Only have one serving and a little portion. A high potassium diet might result in potassium overload, which can impact your heartbeat. Avoid eating tomato sauce, avocado, potato, and banana cream pie at the same meal as your heart cannot handle the high potassium levels.

If you're unfamiliar with the cuisine, don't be afraid to ask about the components. Ask your server if they will make your food without salt. Always remember that you are the consumer, and enjoy!

IMPORTANT TIPS TO NOTE WHEN EATING OUT

Going on a renal-friendly diet does not mean giving up the thrill of dining out. In fact, with the appropriate knowledge and a few clever tactics, you may eat tasty meals without jeopardizing your kidney function. The following is a guide to navigating the dining scene with confidence and choosing choices that are consistent with your renal diet goals.

From interpreting menu options to asking for personalized changes, we'll look at essential methods that will allow you to enjoy restaurant experiences without losing flavor or nutritional balance.

TIPS FOR EATING OUT WITH CKD.

- Plan ahead. When you know you'll be eating at a restaurant or a social gathering, it's crucial to plan ahead. Plan your meals for the day so you can avoid items heavy in salt, potassium, or protein early in the day.
- Contact the host or the restaurant. Inquire with the host or hostess about the planned cuisine. This is an excellent method to talk about nutrition and even offer techniques to reduce sodium in a meal. If you communicate with the restaurant ahead of time, they may prepare lower-sodium meals or recommend other options to match your needs.

- Preview the menu. Most restaurants offer a webpage with their menus, allowing you to organize your day and ensure your nutritional needs are satisfied. Knowing what you're going to eat ahead of time may make you feel more at ease about eating out.

Balanced Plate

You should be mindful of portion sizes and keep your dish balanced. Your plate should be balanced in this way:

- Half of your plate should be vegetables.
- Grains like rice, pasta, and potatoes should make up one-quarter of your dish.
- Protein should account for one-quarter of your dish, including lean meat, fish, chicken, and tofu.

Sodium Tips

- Read the nutrition information on the menu and aim for 700 mg of salt per serving. If you're having something rich in salt, ask for a half dish, split with a buddy, or get a takeout container and take half home to enjoy later.
- Choose fresh foods wherever possible. Foods that are breaded or have sauces will contain more salt.
- Don't add salt to the table.

Protein Tips

- Use your hand to estimate the size of a serving. A palm-size serving contains roughly 2.5 ounces of protein. When determining a portion of beans, peas, or legumes, a fist equals around one cup.
- Request a half serving of protein, or share it with a friend. You can also take half home for another supper the following day.
- If you are limiting your protein consumption, keep in mind that some items, such as cheeses and sauces, may include extra protein; you may be able to substitute or request foods without the extra sauces.

Potassium Tips

If you're on a low-potassium diet, keep in mind that picking meals with lower potassium levels and portion sizes is critical. If you intend to dine out, pick low-potassium items earlier in the day.

This will allow you to eat meals that are not as low in potassium while eating out, providing you with some flexibility.

The following vegetables are lower in potassium:

- Arugula
- String beans (green/yellow)
- Broccoli
- Cabbage
- Cauliflower
- Cucumber
- Eggplant
- Kale
- Leeks
- Lettuce
- Onion
- peppers, and bell
- Radish
- Spaghetti Squash
- Snow peas.
- Turnip
- Watercress
- Zucchini

Tips for Managing Phosphorus

- Phosphorus is utilized as an ingredient in meals, and you may not always have nutritional information that indicates phosphorus has been added. An excellent advice is to buy fresher foods with less phosphorus added.
- When it comes to dessert, choose one that is simple to make and has less hidden phosphorus as an ingredient.
- Share dessert with someone.
- Choose a dessert that is kidney-friendly and low in phosphorus. The following are good options: Fruit, sorbet, angel food cake, apple or lemon pound cake, sugar cookies, shortbread cookies, pies, and cobblers prepared with apples, berries, or lemon.

Eating out can be beneficial for those with CKD as it provides a change from making meals at home and allows for socialization with loved ones. However, don't be scared to express your dietary demands and ask questions. After all, your health comes first, and adhering to dietary limitations is part of that!

FAST FOODS

While this is my least favorite option for eating out, I recognize that because it is so easily available, quick, and inexpensive, many will eat it. If you are accustomed to eating fast food frequently, I recommend you begin cutting back and making healthier options. While fast food is

166

high in salt, phosphorus, bad fats, processed meats, and calories and sugar, there are healthier options available, especially if you are on dialysis. Below are some superior alternatives to a few popular options.

STARBUCKS

Starbucks is the world's largest coffee business, and many people make it a morning routine. Drink sizes typically vary from tall (12 oz) to venti (20 oz), but there is a short (8 oz) option available - great! You should stay away from Frappuccinos. They contain between 37g and 83g of sugar, depending on the size!

Your best bet:

Drinks. Choose Short (8 oz) or Tall (12 oz) based on your fluid limit.

- Coffee: Caffè Americano (hot or iced)
- Shot of espresso, Espresso Macchiato, Cappuccino, and Caffè Latte with almond or coconut milk, available hot or chilled.
- Chai, Black, Green, or Herbal Tea
- Chai Tea Latte has a lot of sugar, therefore get a short size and a single pump chai with almond or coconut milk.
- Matcha Green Tea Latte. Also heavy in sugar, so keep it short and use plant-based milk.
- Cold or Nitro Cold Brew Coffee

Breakfast (Avoid wraps and breakfast sandwiches, as most contain more than 1000 mg of salt).

- Egg bites made with kale and portobello mushrooms. While not the best, it is a better option than breakfast sandwiches and other egg bites.
- Hearty Blueberry Oatmeal (without dried fruit and nuts)
- Sprouted grain or cinnamon raisin bagel, served with cream cheese.
- Butter croissant
- Petite vanilla bean scones

Lunch and snacks (avoid sandwiches; most contain more than 1000 mg of salt).

- PB&J Protein Box (without the chocolate-covered raisins)
- Egg and Cheddar Protein Box

- Prosnax gala/green apples, egg, white cheddar cheese, and almonds/cashews. Snack Box (the lowest salt option among the boxes)
- Butter gourmet popcorn.
- Hippeas
- That's It: Apple + Blueberry Bar
- Blueberry and Oatmeal Jammy Sammy

SUBWAY

Subway is the largest sandwich chain in the USA. You would assume Subway would be healthier than the other fast food options, but there aren't many kidney-friendly selections. Most of their 6-inch sandwiches have over 1000 mg of sodium. According to their ingredient list, all of their meat/protein selections contain phosphate additions except for the tuna salad and meatballs; nevertheless, the meatballs are drenched in marinara sauce and rich in sodium and potassium, making them an unsuitable choice for dialysis patients. Avoid all wraps and breakfast products, as they are high in salt. To reduce sodium/potassium content, avoid adding chips and keep bananas, jalapeño peppers, pickles, black olives, and tomatoes.

Your best bets:

- Tuna sandwich, protein bowl, or salad
- Veggie Delight Sandwich with Swiss Cheese.
- Oven-roasted chicken sandwich or salad.
- Turkey breast sandwich or salad.
- Sweet onion chicken teriyaki sandwich or salad.
- Fresh prepared iced tea and Dasani water.
- Applesauce

McDONALD'S

McDonald's is the world's most popular fast-food restaurant chain, with about 40,000 locations worldwide. Unfortunately, there are numerous terrible options for dialysis patients. All of the breakfast sausages contain salt and sugar, the biscuits and pancakes contain salt and phosphate additives, the hamburger patties contain salt, the pickles contain salt and potassium sorbate (a preservative), the ketchup contains high fructose corn syrup and salt, the hotcake syrup contains

168

high fructose corn syrup, sugar, and potassium sorbate, the processed cheese, and so on. *Here are a few guidelines to help you make a better dinner choice:*

- Do not request cheese, pickles, ketchup, or mustard (or on the side so you may regulate the quantity).
- The majority of the breakfast meal contains high levels of salt and phosphorus. Avoid hotcakes, McGriddles, hash browns, most breakfast sandwiches (particularly those with biscuits), and sausage burritos.
- Avoid french fries (rich in potassium and salt).
- The majority of McDonald's desserts, shakes, smoothies, and drinks are poor choices.

Your best bets:

- Breakfast: Fruit and Maple Oatmeal; Egg McMuffin without Canadian bacon.
- Coffee, tea, Americano, and Espresso (small = 12 oz).
- Hamburger Filet-O-Fish. Ask for tartar sauce on the side (it contains salt and potassium sorbate).
- McChicken (contains phosphate additions but is low in salt).
- Garden salad McNuggets with ranch or honey mustard. Reminder: This includes more than 500mg of salt, therefore if taken with a sandwich, your lunch may easily exceed 1000 mg of sodium. Only choose if you do not intend to have a sandwich or burger.
- Sides: apple slices and a pineapple stick.
- Dessert: apple pie.
- Drinks (small = 16 oz/2 cups): iced tea, water, Sprite, or 12 oz apple juice. Add plenty of ice and savor leisurely.

KFC

KFC (Kentucky Fried Chicken) is the fourth-largest fast-food restaurant chain. I worked hard to come up with excellent bets, but I believe this is one of the worst fast food selections available. The chicken is of poor quality, with excessive salt, MSG, and phosphate additions. Eating just one grilled chicken drumstick contains almost 1100 mg of sodium, and that doesn't include sides like high phosphorus/sodium biscuits, mac and cheese, mashed potatoes and gravy, or BBQ baked beans.

I would avoid most of their menu items except for the following sides: green beans, sweet corn, corn on the cob, coleslaw, macaroni salad, side salad, and apple turnover. Sorry, there aren't many recommended selections!

TACO BELL

If you ask me, this is a bad imitation of Mexican food. While not the most popular fast food chain, I thought I'd include it for variety. The majority of menu items contain high levels of potassium, sodium, and phosphorus, leaving few kidney-friendly options. Their seasoned beef contains phosphate chemicals, and just one normal bean burrito has 1000 mg of sodium.

Even without red sauce and cheddar cheese, it has 800 mg of salt. Their cheese sauce includes phosphate and potassium additions. The majority of the breakfast menu, including all burritos and quesadillas, power menu bowls, quesalupas, crunch wraps, and nachos, is not good.

The following are your best bets.

- 1-2 Crunchy Tacos with no cheese, tomatoes, or additional hot sauce. This is an excellent opportunity to utilize your homemade salt-free spicy sauce!
- One soft taco without cheese, tomatoes, or hot sauce. There is an option to add rice. Note that the flour tortilla contains phosphorus additions.
- Chalupa or Black Bean Chalupa served with lettuce, onions, and sour cream
- Chicken Chipotle Melt
- A side of chips with nacho cheese sauce. Not the healthiest option, and the cheese sauce contains phosphate additions, however, it has an appropriate sodium content per serving.
- Sweets: Cinnabon delights and cinnamon twists.
- Drinks (small=16 oz/2 cups): coffee, iced coffee, and water. Most fountain beverages include more than 50 grams of sugar, and Brisk iced tea, especially when unsweetened, contains phosphoric acid (a phosphorus ingredient).

Whew! I believe we covered a wide range of eating-out possibilities. From Asian to Taco Bell, you should be able to make the most dialysis-friendly options. While it is preferable and healthier to prepare meals at home, there will always be situations when you must dine out. Just remember the Tips & Tricks and make sure you have your phosphorus binders with you!

I WISH YOU HAPPY, HEALTHY EATING WITH NO REGRETS!

CHAPTER 14

FREQUENTLY ASKED QUESTIONS (FAQs)

As we navigate through the complexities of renal health and the intricacies of a renal-friendly diet, questions often arise. In this comprehensive FAQ section, we address some of the most commonly asked questions, providing you with valuable insights and practical solutions.

Here are a few questions you can expect to find answers to:

1. Is a transplant operation possible??
2. Is Anaemia linked to Kidney failure?
3. What is end stage renal disease?
4. Is there a cure for CKD or ESRD?
5. What is dialysis?

And so many more.......

ACCESSING DETAILED ANSWERS:

For an in-depth exploration of these questions and more, **SCAN THE QR CODES BELOW**. These resources are designed to complement the information in this chapter, offering you a wealth of knowledge to support your renal wellness journey. These links will take you to an external resource that is in no way associated with the author or this book in general. The information in these resources have been carefully reviewed by legal practitioners.

We understand that your journey to optimal kidney health is unique, and these FAQs aim to address concerns that resonate with many individuals navigating similar paths. Your questions matter, and by providing accessible resources, we aim to empower you with the information you need to make informed decisions about your renal health.

Feel free to reach out with additional questions or explore the provided links for a deeper dive into the world of renal well-being. Your proactive approach to understanding and managing your health is commendable, and we're here to support you every step of the way.

CONCLUSION

As we conclude this insightful journey through the realms of renal health and the nuances of a kidney-friendly lifestyle, it's time to reflect on the milestones achieved and look forward to the road ahead. In this concluding chapter, we celebrate not only the progress made but also the inspiring success stories of those who have embraced the principles of a renal-friendly diet.

Celebrating Progress:

Your commitment to understanding and implementing a renal-friendly lifestyle has undoubtedly led to positive changes. Whether it's mastering the art of meal preparation, deciphering nutrition labels with ease, or confidently making choices that support kidney health, every step is a testament to your dedication. Take a moment to acknowledge the progress made, no matter how small; each achievement contributes to the larger tapestry of well-being.

Encouragement for the Journey Ahead:

The road to optimal kidney health is ongoing, and as you navigate the twists and turns, remember that progress is a continuous journey. Embrace each day as an opportunity to make choices that align with your health goals. Let setbacks be stepping stones to growth, and successes be the fuel that propels you forward. As you venture into the future, may your commitment to renal well-being be a source of strength and resilience.

A Heartfelt Thank You:

Before we bid adieu, a sincere thank you for entrusting this guide with your renal health journey. Your curiosity, dedication, and perseverance have illuminated the pages of this book, turning it into a collaborative exploration of well-being. Remember, you're not alone in this journey; a supportive community stands alongside you, ready to inspire, share insights, and celebrate successes.

As you close this chapter, may the principles ingrained in these pages accompany you on your continued path to thriving renal health. Your commitment to understanding, embracing, and celebrating the intricacies of a renal-friendly lifestyle is a commendable feat. Here's to your health, your journey, and the vibrant chapters that lie ahead.

Wishing you strength, joy, and continued success on your renal wellness adventure.

WARM REGARDS,

JUANITA SCOTT.

AUTHOR, FATTY LIVER DIET COOKBOOK FOR SENIORS AND BEGINNERS

COOKING CONVERSION CHARTS

MEASUREMENTS

CUPS	OUNCES	MILLILITERS	TABLESPOONS
8 cups	64 oz	1895 mil	128
6 cups	48 oz	1420 mil	96
5 cups	40 oz	1120 mil	80
4 cups	32 oz	960 mil	64
2 cup	16 oz	480 mil	32
1 cup	8 oz	240 mil	16
¾ cup	6 oz	177 mil	12
⅔ cup	5 oz	158 mil	11
½ cup	4 oz	118 mil	8
⅜ cup	3 oz	90 mil	6
⅓ cup	2.5 oz	79 mil	5.5
¼ cup	2 oz	59 mil	4
⅛ cup	1 oz	30 mil	3
1/16 cup	½ oz	15 mil	1

TEMPERATURE

FAHRENHEIT	CELCIUS
100 °F	37 °C
150 °F	65 °C
200 °F	93 °C
250 °F	121 °C
300 °F	150 °C
325 °F	160 °C
350 °F	180 °C
375 °F	190 °C
400 °F	200 °C
425 °F	220 °C
450 °F	230 °C
500 °F	260 °C
525 °F	274 °C
550 °F	288 °C

WEIGHT

IMPERIAL	METRIC
½ oz	15 g
1 oz	29 g
2 oz	57 g
3 oz	85 g
4 oz	113 g
5 oz	141 g
6 oz	170 g
8 oz	227 g
10 oz	283 g
12 oz	340 g
13 oz	369 g
14 oz	397 g
15 oz	425 g
1 lb	453 g

MY GIFT TO YOU

Dearest Reader,

As we come to an end of this fulfilling trip, I would like to express my deep thanks to you. I've prepared not just one special bonus but three special bonuses for you as a thank you (I always keep my promises). These gifts are in forms of PDFs. These PDFs are additional resources to guide you on your journey to a amazing health.

To get your bonus:

1. Scan the QR code that's right here in the middle of this page to obtain your bonus.
2. You'll be directed to a unique download page where your exclusive bonus is waiting for you.

SCAN THESE QR CODES TO GET YOUR BONUS!

This book was inspired by your passion for living a better lifestyle, and I'm excited to provide you with these extra tools.

Again, I appreciate that you selected the "Renal Diet Cookbook for Beginners 2024." May you have many satisfying and life-changing meals on your path to wellness.

A DEEP REQUEST

Dearest Reader,

I hope you've had the chance to dive into "The Renal Diet Cookbook for Beginners 2024." Your opinion matters greatly, and I would be honored to hear your thoughts. Your honest reviews play a crucial role in helping others discover the benefits of this comprehensive guide.

Whether you've tried the recipes, followed the meal plan, or simply enjoyed the insights shared, your feedback is invaluable. Please take a moment to share your thoughts on platforms like Amazon, Goodreads, or any other platform where you obtained your copy.

Your reviews not only guide future readers but also contribute to the ongoing conversation about kidney health. Thank you for being a part of this journey, and I look forward to hearing from you.

RECOMMENDED READING

Dearest Esteemed Reader,

I trust you're enjoying "The Renal Diet Cookbook for Beginners 2024" and finding it beneficial on your health journey. If you've been inspired by my approach to wellness, I'd like to introduce you to another valuable resource in my collection — "Fatty Liver for Seniors and Beginners."

This insightful guide is tailored to support individuals navigating the complexities of fatty liver concerns, offering practical advice and a range of accessible strategies for seniors and beginners alike.

Explore more from my authorship by visiting my author page, where you'll discover a wealth of information designed to empower you on your path to better health. To visit my author page, all you need to do is scan the QR code below. The QR code will take you straight to my author page.

SCAN HERE!

Thank you for your continued support and trust in my commitment to providing comprehensive health resources.

Best regards,

Juanita Scott.

INDEX

MY 4-WEEK

Meal Plan

BELONGS TO

Bonus
MEAL PLAN

Week :

Date :

MONDAY

Breakfast	Fruit and Oat Pancakes
Lunch	Egg White & Pepper Omelets
Dinner	Minestrone Soup
Desserts	Poor Man's Cake

TUESDAY

Breakfast	Bell Pepper and Feta Crustless Quiche
Lunch	Fresh Fruit Compote
Dinner	Crispy Baked Cauliflower Wings
Desserts	Butterscotch Bars

WEDNESDAY

Breakfast	Mexican Brunch Eggs
Lunch	Cilantro Lime Cod
Dinner	Vegetable and Tofu Stir-Fry
Desserts	Apple Pie

THURSDAY

Breakfast	French Toast
Lunch	Ginger Spiced Lamb Chops
Dinner	Garlic Mashed Potatoes
Desserts	Yellow Cake

FRIDAY

Breakfast	Egg Sandwich
Lunch	Shrimp in Garlic Sauce (High Protein)
Dinner	Baked Tilapia Filets Gremolata
Desserts	Margarita Freezer Pie

SATURDAY

Breakfast	Asparagus & Swiss Cheese Frittata
Lunch	Ratatouille
Dinner	Quinoa Dressing
Desserts	Pineapple Angel Cake

SUNDAY

Breakfast	Blueberry Peanut Butter Oatmeal
Lunch	Beef & Sweet Potato Burgers
Dinner	Grilled Marinated Chicken
Desserts	Fruit Pizza

WATER INTAKE

MONDAY								
TUESDAY								
WEDNESDAY								
THURSDAY								
FRIDAY								
SATURDAY								
SUNDAY								

Bonus
MEAL PLAN

MONDAY

Breakfast	Egg & Rice Muffins
Lunch	Zucchini Bread
Dinner	Spinach and Feta Stuffed Chicken Breast
Desserts	Fiesta Tilapia Ceviche

TUESDAY

Breakfast	Italian Eggs and Peppers
Lunch	Zucchini Bread
Dinner	Linguine with Garlic and Shrimp
Desserts	Fruit Crispies

WEDNESDAY

Breakfast	Spicy Tofu Scrambler
Lunch	Lemon and Berry Bread
Dinner	Grilled Marinated Chicken
Desserts	Keto Brownie

THURSDAY

Breakfast	Spicy Tofu Scrambler
Lunch	Golden Potato Croquettes
Dinner	Quinoa Dressing
Desserts	Apple Pie

FRIDAY

Breakfast	Cottage Cheese Pancakes
Lunch	Thai Chicken Curry
Dinner	Roasted Turkey Breast with Salt-Free Herb Seasoning
Desserts	Butterscotch Bars

SATURDAY

Breakfast	Spicy Cornbread
Lunch	Shish Kebabs
Dinner	Quinoa Dressing
Desserts	Margarita Freezer Pie

SUNDAY

Breakfast	Vegetarian Summer Rolls
Lunch	Creamy Shrimp and Broccoli Fettuccine
Dinner	Baked Tilapia Filets Gremolata
Desserts	Yellow Cake

WATER INTAKE

MONDAY	⊔ ⊔ ⊔ ⊔ ⊔ ⊔ ⊔ ⊔
TUESDAY	⊔ ⊔ ⊔ ⊔ ⊔ ⊔ ⊔ ⊔
WEDNESDAY	⊔ ⊔ ⊔ ⊔ ⊔ ⊔ ⊔ ⊔
THURSDAY	⊔ ⊔ ⊔ ⊔ ⊔ ⊔ ⊔ ⊔
FRIDAY	⊔ ⊔ ⊔ ⊔ ⊔ ⊔ ⊔ ⊔
SATURDAY	⊔ ⊔ ⊔ ⊔ ⊔ ⊔ ⊔ ⊔
SUNDAY	⊔ ⊔ ⊔ ⊔ ⊔ ⊔ ⊔ ⊔

Bonus
MEAL PLAN

MONDAY

Breakfast	Buckwheat Pancakes
Lunch	Gobi Curry
Dinner	Garlic Mashed Potatoes
Desserts	Blueberry Peach Crisp

TUESDAY

Breakfast	Cheesesteak Quiche
Lunch	Stir-Fried Garlic Green Beans with Toasted Almonds
Dinner	Quinoa Dressing
Desserts	Warm Bread Pudding

WEDNESDAY

Breakfast	40-Second Omelet
Lunch	Baked Sea Bass and Roasted Red Pepper
Dinner	Grilled Marinated Chicken
Desserts	Margarita Freezer Pie

THURSDAY

Breakfast	Sour Cream Apple Bread
Lunch	Vegan Bolognese Sauce
Dinner	Shrimp Quesadilla
Desserts	Apple Crisp

FRIDAY

Breakfast	Strawberry Bread
Lunch	Roasted Asparagus and Wild Mushroom Stew
Dinner	Linguine with Garlic and Shrimp
Desserts	Butterscotch Bars

SATURDAY

Breakfast	Italian Apple Fritters
Lunch	Creamy Shrimp and Broccoli Fettuccine
Dinner	Baked Tilapia Filets Gremolata
Desserts	Yellow Cake

SUNDAY

Breakfast	Green Beans with Turnips
Lunch	Tortilla Beef Roll-Ups (High Protein)
Dinner	Roasted Turkey Breast with Salt-Free Herb Seasoning
Desserts	Margarita Freezer Pie

WATER INTAKE

MONDAY								
TUESDAY								
WEDNESDAY								
THURSDAY								
FRIDAY								
SATURDAY								
SUNDAY								

Bonus
MEAL PLAN

MONDAY

Breakfast	Cottage Cheese Pancakes
Lunch	Mediterranean Lamb Patties
Dinner	Spinach and Feta Stuffed Chicken Breast
Desserts	Fruit Pizza

TUESDAY

Breakfast	Egg & Avocado Bake
Lunch	Stir-Fried Garlic Green Beans with Toasted Almonds
Dinner	Quinoa Dressing
Desserts	Gingerbread Apple Cobbler

WEDNESDAY

Breakfast	Buckwheat Pancakes
Lunch	Kidney Bean Salad
Dinner	Grilled Marinated Chicken
Desserts	Home-Style Vanilla Ice Cream

THURSDAY

Breakfast	Apple Spice Muffins
Lunch	Roasted Turkey Breast with Salt-Free Herb Seasoning
Dinner	Linguine with Garlic and Shrimp
Desserts	Butterscotch Bars

FRIDAY

Breakfast	French Toast
Lunch	Creamy Shrimp and Broccoli Fettuccine
Dinner	Baked Tilapia Filets Gremolata
Desserts	Margarita Freezer Pie

SATURDAY

Breakfast	Cheesesteak Quiche
Lunch	Vegan Bolognese Sauce
Dinner	Baked Sea Bass and Roasted Red Pepper
Desserts	Apple Crisp

SUNDAY

Breakfast	Blueberry Peanut Butter Oatmeal
Lunch	Creamy Shrimp and Broccoli Fettuccine
Dinner	Grilled Marinated Chicken
Desserts	Yellow Cake

WATER INTAKE

MONDAY	
TUESDAY	
WEDNESDAY	
THURSDAY	
FRIDAY	
SATURDAY	
SUNDAY	

www.ingramcontent.com/pod-product-compliance
Lightning Source LLC
Chambersburg PA
CBHW080945290526

45795CB00009B/2923